"How Could I Have Had a Heart Attack? I Watch Doctor Oz!!"

Kim Waldrup

This book is not intended to treat or diagnose any medical condition. Nor is it a substitute for your physician's care and does not support or endorse any product, procedure or company. It is recommended that you consult your physician before making any changes to your current medication or treatment.

Front Cover Photo by Kirk Voclain Photography,
Houma, Louisiana 70360

Copyright © 2011, Kim Waldrup
All rights reserved, including the right to reproduce, store, or transmit this book or any portion thereof in any form whatsoever without written permission, except for brief quotations embodied in critical articles and reviews.
ISBN: 978-1505366143

This book is dedicated to my wonderful family and friends. I will never forget the love and kindness that you have shown me through this journey. You have all played a major role in my recovery, and are the reasons for my heart to keep beating. I thank each and every one of you from the bottom of my mended heart.

In memory of all those who have lost their fight in the battle against heart disease.

I would like to acknowledge the staff of Cardiovascular Institute of the South and Terrebonne General Medical Center. I offer a heartfelt thank you to all who contributed towards my excellent care and recovery. A *special* thanks goes out to the skilled, caring cath lab team.

I would also like to sincerely thank Siera Martinez, Rose Pitre, Tracy Dorsey and Kacie Woods for their tremendous help with the arduous editing process.

A special thank you to my wonderful son-in-law, Chris Derish, for all your help, patience and for being my technical advisor.

CHAPTER 1

A heart attack is a serious event. In fact, it can prove to be life changing, if not life ending. Yet, we talk about heart attacks quite casually on a daily basis. We say things like, "I was so angry that I thought I was going to have a heart attack." or "Don't scare me like that! Do you want me to have a heart attack?" Someone will say, "Are you serious?" We glibly reply, "Serious as a heart attack." We say these things nonchalantly in passing, without even giving it a second thought.

There is even the "Hollywood heart attack." We're all familiar with that one. It's the one we see in the movies and on television. Suddenly, the stressed-out business executive winces and shrugs his shoulders forward. He looks uncomfortable as he loosens his tie. In the next frame, he's sweating profusely and looks like he's in agony. He drops his briefcase and firmly clutches the left side of his chest. He then falls to the floor.

There are even comedic skits that portray them. The one imbedded in my mind is the unforgettable recollection from the 1970's. Redd Foxx starred as the character of Fred Sanford. He stumbled, stiff-legged around the room, grasping his chest. He looked upward and uttered those classic words, "It's the big one Lizabeth. I'm coming Lizabeth." Forever engraved in our memories, it always brought a huge roar of laughter. I am smiling now, as I think about it and write this. However, a heart attack is *no* laughing matter! I know this on a personal level.

When we seriously think of a heart attack, what usually comes to our minds? We usually think of someone whom we love that was affected by a heart attack. It could be a husband or father, a dear friend or brother. So, what's the commonality here? They're *all* men! We rarely think of a woman as having a heart attack. I know I really didn't give it much thought, until it happened to me. One purpose of this story is to let you know that women *do* have heart attacks! It's not simply "a man's disease," as once thought.

Statistics show that heart attack is the single leading cause of death for American women. Many women believe that cancer is more of a danger, but this isn't the case. Almost twice as many women in the United States die of heart disease than from all forms of cancer combined. In fact, six times more women die from heart disease than from breast cancer. Women, it seems, also have a worse outcome than men do *after* having a heart attack. They are one and a half times more likely than men are to die in the first year following a heart attack. One reason for this may be that women often delay going to the hospital for treatment when they experience the often-indiscernible onset of symptoms. The sooner proper treatment is initiated the better the prognosis. The problem is, we simply do not equate our symptoms with a heart attack since for years, "heart attack" was just not on our radar. Besides that, we think it's our job to take care of others *first*, and then ourselves. We need to rethink this concept if we want to be around to care for the ones that we love.

You've probably heard that a woman's heart attack is different from that of a man's. I can tell you that you had better believe it. It's different in that a woman's symptoms, much of the time, present in an unconventional manner. I want to tell my story so that my experience may help someone else…maybe even save their life. Perhaps others can learn from my mistakes—now that I realize I've made a lot of them. I don't claim to be an expert; however, I did have a front row seat in this saga. That reality has caused me to gain much insight.

In the interest of truth and accuracy, I will attempt to recreate this event as honestly and in as much detail as possible. I'll not only include the facts, but my own fears and foibles as well. I appreciate *now* that my errors in judgment probably contributed to my heart attack. I'll discuss the physical as well as the emotional impact that a cardiac event can bring. I know personally, that as with any serious event in our lives, it can bring much grief and upheaval. In sharing my story, I hope that I might bring to light not only the symptoms, but also information on what *you* can do personally to protect your own heart. At the very least, if you are a fellow heart attack survivor, you'll know that you're not alone in the things that you are thinking and feeling.

***

I imagine that women may have always had heart attacks, although I'm not actually sure. For whatever reason though, we all have a mind-set that men seem to own the heart attack monopoly. I certainly thought so. After all, in my family, it had been my father and maternal grandfather who had ended up on the short end of the heart attack stick. For this reason, I naturally worried about my husband. I did what most women do. I "actively managed" my husband's health. I saw to it that *he* had his vitamins, ate well, and watched *his* cholesterol. At first, he resisted taking cholesterol medication because of concerns about their side effects, but in time, agreed to take them. He had issues with his blood pressure, which was a concern to me as well. I made sure that *he* took his medicine, watched *his* sodium, and got *his* yearly check-ups. The problem was ... I didn't do *most* of those things for *myself*. After all, as a *woman*, I didn't have to worry as much about those things since most of that applied to men. Men were at the greatest risk for heart related issues, *or so I thought*.

About three weeks before my heart attack I did something that would prove very ironic. I saw an advertisement in the newspaper for a free screening at the local cardiology office. I asked my husband if he would like to attend. He agreed to go, so I made an appointment for *him*, but not myself. His appointment was scheduled for late afternoon, Tuesday, July 26, 2011. Of course, being the dutiful wife and health-care provider/guardian that I was, I accompanied him. When we checked in with the receptionist, she asked if I was participating as well. I told her that I hadn't made an appointment for myself. She told me that there was an opening if I'd be interested in joining in. I thought, "Why not?"

The screening included several different tests. The tests offered were a glucose reading, total cholesterol check, body mass index, and ankle-brachial index (ABI). In this test, blood pressure is measured in the arms and legs simultaneously and a computer comparison is then made of the pressures. This test is a diagnostic tool to screen for peripheral artery disease.

Peripheral artery disease refers to a buildup of plaque in any area of the body, other than the heart. It's often an indicator of coronary artery disease. That was the main reason I had signed my husband up for the screening. I wanted to be certain that his heart was in good shape.

Each test was set up at different stations. We started through the maze. First, it was the glucose check. My glucose level was 105. That wasn't bad for late in the afternoon and after a small meal. I had just eaten a small hamburger about 45 minutes earlier. Next, it was the cholesterol test. I was taken aback when the test revealed a whopping 290-total cholesterol. The technician commented on the fact that it was very high. I quickly offered an excuse. I explained that I had just eaten a hamburger, which was probably the reason it was so high. I have however, come to realize that I can be quite adept at using excuses to dismiss things I don't have an answer to or that I just don't want to confront.

The truth was my cholesterol was *usually* high. For the past six years or so, my total cholesterol numbers had been somewhere between 230 and 240. In my mind, I didn't think those numbers were excessively high, at least not high enough that I should be *overly* concerned about them. My family doctor had wanted to prescribe cholesterol medication, but I resisted. I had heard so many bad things about those types of medications. There were numerous side effects that I simply didn't want to deal with. In view of that, I decided I would improve my diet, and I did. In fact, I would be extra careful *right before* blood work. I would watch what I ate more cautiously with the hope of altering the test results. I would eat oatmeal as if it were going out of style. I also tried natural remedies in order to improve my numbers, although I wasn't always consistent with this method. Sometimes ... it *actually* worked! When it did, the doctor would back off on trying to get me to take the cholesterol medication. The problem was I didn't eat like that all the time. I will say in my defense, I thought that we ate better than most people did. I was well aware of the principles of good nutrition and I tried to apply them, by feeding my family good, healthy meals.

Now, as I reflect on this method, I'm not sure who I *thought* I was fooling. Nonetheless, I realize in retrospect that I was only fooling myself. Still, at the time, I just didn't want to hear it because I thought *I* knew better. I can now appreciate that to ignore the facts do not change them. I should have listened to my doctor and been more consistent in my self-treatment. Of course hindsight, after all, is 20/20.

Let's go back to the health screening. The next station was for a BMI (body mass index). According to my numbers, I was within normal range for a female in my age group. That surprised me, because I knew that I was at least twenty-five pounds overweight. The nurse who was in charge of the BMI, noticed that my cholesterol numbers were high. She asked me if I was a patient at the clinic. I smiled and quickly responded that I wasn't.

She smiled back, nodded her head and liltingly replied, "*You will be.*" Little did either of us know at that point in time—that in less than three weeks, her prophecy that day *would* come true.

I next went for the ABI and my results for that test were normal. At the completion of the screening, we were able to review the results with one of the cardiologists, Dr. Anil Chagarlamudi. (Initially most patients and staff had difficulty pronouncing his last name, so now everyone just calls him Dr. Anil.) He told us everything looked good, *with the exception* of my cholesterol. He urged me to get it under control. I promised that I would. I thought then that I might even consider cholesterol medications. My husband had been taking them, and he didn't appear to be experiencing any problems. My husband and I left happy and hand in hand. We thought we were good to go. Little did we know that in as little as three days, the start of a declining chain of events would be set into motion.

CHAPTER 2

Friday Afternoon, July 29, 2011

That afternoon I felt tired and decided to lay down for a nap. You may be thinking that extreme fatigue is one of the signs before a heart attack. You're right, that's certainly true. However, this was not out of the ordinary for me. I have been a low-energy person ever since I can remember. As a child when I complained, my mother would tell me, "You were born tired." I have always had to push myself in order to get things accomplished. I have hypothyroidism, and had been taking medication for this condition for about fourteen years. About a year earlier, I was diagnosed with Hashimoto's disease. Hashimoto's is an autoimmune disorder that affects the thyroid. I was under the care of an endocrinologist and both of these conditions were under control, to my knowledge. I used these conditions as my "go-to" excuses for the reasons I felt tired much of the time.

Napping was, and *is* something I've always really enjoyed, so I was looking forward to my afternoon catnap. As I was trying to drift off to sleep, I noticed a pain in my left shoulder blade. The pain went up into my neck as well. That really didn't strike me as odd though. I've had neck pain for a long time. In fact, I'd been in a car accident and had a whiplash injury about thirty-five years ago. The discomfort was something I had become accustomed to over the years. It wasn't constant, but would come and go. However, in the past few months I had noticed that it did seem to be hurting more frequently. As for the shoulder pain, I had undergone shoulder surgery two years earlier. Therefore, I was no stranger to shoulder pain. I assumed the pain I felt that afternoon were from these old injuries. My reasoning on this matter seemed plausible to me at the time. On the other hand, was I perhaps just looking for a reasonable excuse ... *again*?

This time, the pain was more in the shoulder blade, in the mid-back. Normally when it hurts, it hurts in the shoulder joint where it connects to the arm. Not this time though, but still, I dismissed it. Then something odd happened. My left arm started hurting on the upper portion, and on the lower portion, there was numbness. It was disconcerting, albeit brief. A fleeting thought went through my mind, "I hope I'm not having a heart attack."

I was certainly familiar with the whole "arm numbness thing" connected to heart attacks. Over the years, I'd read several articles about heart attacks. I had even saved some of them. I wanted to be aware, just to be on the safe side. Would you believe there was even a checklist on the side of my refrigerator from the American Heart Association? It was a list of the warning signs to look for. My mother had always been concerned and interested in matters related to health. She impressed upon me that this was important, so I endeavored to stay informed. I felt confident that I was. The numbness lasted just a short time, maybe 20-30 seconds, and then went away. I thought it could have just been my arm falling asleep. The shoulder pain continued, but that too, came and went. Still, I ignored it. I have since learned that the word "ignore" comes from the same Latin root word as "ignorance." Interesting isn't it?

On Sunday, I was talking with a friend and her husband. He asked me how I was doing. I told him, my back and neck were hurting me, relating to them that it had been hurting on and off since Friday.

I next revealed to my friend the incident of the numbness in my arm saying, "It was kind of odd. I thought for a moment that I was having a heart attack."

She asked if I had gone to the doctor and I replied I hadn't because it was a Friday afternoon and the likelihood of getting an appointment before the weekend was slim. I assured her that the numbness didn't last for long and jokingly said, "I guess it wasn't a heart attack or I would be dead by now." We laughed it off.

Monday, August 2, 2011

My mother had a friend visiting from Florida and she wanted to go to the French Quarter for lunch. No trip to South Louisiana would be complete without doing so. We live about sixty miles from the beautiful, historic city of New Orleans—a city widely known for its fun, food and music. Its charm and charisma make it a wonderful place to visit. The unique architecture of the French Quarter is spectacular and reminiscent of an old European city. To preserve the French and Spanish influences of the past, buildings have been carefully restored. Today, it's a colorful blend of old and new. New Orleans is an extremely resilient city as well, that has bounced back even after the devastation of hurricane Katrina.

That was our plan for Monday. We were going to have lunch in the French Quarter. My older daughter lives in a suburb of New Orleans and she was planning to come along with us as well, it was going to be a fun "girls' day out." Parking in the French Quarter can be a nightmare. For this reason, we decided to take the Algiers ferry across the Mississippi River. It's a short ride and as a bonus, you can see the beautiful view of the shoreline. The French Quarter is situated along a giant curve or crescent in the Mississippi River. New Orleans, also called the Crescent City, gained its nickname because of this. Everything in the French Quarter is in close proximity, so walking is not a problem. It's actually more enjoyable because you get to see all the treasures in the little shops along the way. My daughter and my mother's friend stayed on deck. My mother and I went inside where it was cool for the ride, since it was a very hot day.

We docked and started towards the café for lunch, a quaint little café that is a favorite of ours. They serve the best muffulettas in the Quarter. If you are not acquainted with the muffuletta, allow me to elaborate. It is a *mammoth* sandwich that is named for the round Sicilian bun on which it is assembled. Legend has it that it was originally created in New Orleans by an Italian grocer. It is comprised of a large sesame-seeded bun with layers of provolone and traditional Italian cold cuts of salami, mortadella, and capicola. Finally, it is topped with a special, tasty olive salad mix that makes your mouth water.

We were en route to the café and my shoulders and neck started to hurt. They felt tight and tense and as we continued to walk, the pain strengthened. I started to feel a little out of breath as well. As I said, it was a very hot August day and there was no shade along the way. Between the heat and the mounting pain, I was instantly sorry that I had come. I realized that this day was going to be a long, difficult, day due to the way I was feeling. Besides that, I didn't want to ruin the day of fun for my companions.

I had even thought ahead that morning. I had ditched my gigantic purse in favor of a much smaller, lighter one. As we walked, I was hurting more and more. I finally told my daughter how much pain I was experiencing. I guess I didn't look like I was feeling well, because she offered to carry my purse. She wanted me to stop to rest, but I refused because we were in the hot sun and there was no place to sit except the filthy sidewalk. *That* was out of the question for this germaphobe! We walked a little further until we got to a covered area where I leaned up against the building to rest and cool off. My daughter had ibuprofen in her purse and she offered it to me for the pain. So, I quickly grabbed three and downed them with her water. I would learn later that my companions were all very concerned about me because they feared a heart attack. I rested a few minutes longer and then resumed walking toward the café.

We finally reached our destination. We went in and ordered our food. It arrived quickly, and was *absolutely* delicious! The café was cool and I drank a large glass of iced tea. I figured that the ibuprofen had kicked in because I was able to relax during lunch. My mother wanted me to put ice on my neck. She is a firm believer in ice therapy. My mother's friend had a zipper bag in her purse and the server was kind enough to fill it with ice for me before we left. I was wearing a top with a hoodie that day; I put the ice bag in the hoodie and pulled the drawstring tight. It wasn't exactly a fashion statement, but it worked in a pinch. I felt much better at this point, completely back to normal.

We left the café and headed toward Café du Monde. Café du Monde is world famous for its beignets and café au lait. That is all they sell, and they are divine! If you've never eaten beignets, they are these light, tender, fluffy confections. They're made from yeast-based dough that's cut into squares and are then fried and topped with copious amounts of powdered sugar. Everyone ends up with a powdered sugar mustache and your lap dusted in white powder. (Note: *Never* wear black or navy when eating beignets.) Some uninformed people call them donuts, but that *does not* do them justice. As we started walking again, the pain in my neck and shoulders returned. It was not quite as bad as it had been earlier. I figured that the ibuprofen was taking the edge off. We finally got to Café du Monde. We each ordered beignets and coffee. They were, as expected, messy *and* wonderful. Again, after sitting and resting, I felt better.

Now, we had to take the long walk back to the ferry and I didn't know how I was going to make it. By this time, the ice in the zipper bag had for the most part, melted. There was a pharmacy nearby, I stopped in and bought an instant ice pack. As we started back, we realized that we were near the river front streetcar pick-up station. Everyone agreed to ride the streetcar instead of walking. I was *so* thankful. At least that would shorten my walking time. I noticed that it was while I was walking, that it seemed to be when my neck and shoulders ached most. We finally made it to the ferry and then the car. My mother and I set out for home. I felt just fine on the ride home. My pain had subsided, *for now*.

CHAPTER 3

Tuesday, August 3, 2011

The next day I was in pain again. I made an appointment to see my chiropractor. I thought he might be able to give me some much-needed relief, so I went to see him that afternoon. I felt better while he was adjusting my neck and back. The relief nevertheless was short-lived. The pain would come and go as I *pushed* myself to function, hoping that it would improve.

The next two days were more of the same. The following day, Friday, August 5, my husband and I had made plans to go to a water park with our daughters and grandson. The water park is about two hours away from our home. This is something we do nearly every summer and the summer was almost gone. I really wanted to back out because of the way I had been feeling, but I resisted the urge to stay home since this had been a family tradition for many years.

We left early that morning. I told my husband all I planned to do that day was to go to the Lazy Lagoon. He liked that idea too. Surely sitting in an inner tube going around and around would be *nice* and *relaxing*. That was just what I needed. When we arrived, my neck wasn't hurting at the time. My husband and I started our lazy day on the Lazy Lagoon. This was going to be our day to unwind. There is no exertion involved, just floating. However, by the time we got off after only one trip around, my neck and shoulders were so tight with tremendous pain that intensified with only a fraction of movement. I didn't understand why I was hurting so much.

As we were getting out of the water, the kids were coming to meet us. For their first ride, they had opted for a more challenging one than we had.

"Don't freak out" my daughter started—as if I wouldn't freak out to a sentence like *that*— "but I passed out for a few seconds when I got to the top of the ride."

I immediately questioned her about what had happened. It was another very hot, typical South Louisiana summer day. I was at first concerned that her passing out could be heat related. Then she began telling me that she had run up the steps very quickly and said when she got to the top of the platform, she suddenly felt very sleepy, started yawning and blacked out. I knew she'd eaten a good breakfast less than two hours earlier; therefore, I ruled out that it was blood sugar related. Still, I just didn't know what the problem was. Of course I was concerned, I was her mother. She assured me that she was fine. Despite her telling me this, I asked her if she wanted to go home. She said she didn't. I was hoping that she would say she did. I was hurting so much and *I really* did want to go home.

My husband and I found two deck chairs in the semi-shade. I hoped that resting would make me feel better. It did not! The pain was extreme and I was miserable.

After some time, I told my husband that I truly *needed* to leave. The kids were in a separate car, so they decided to stay a little longer. I hated to leave, especially with what had happened earlier with my daughter. We started out for home. I relaxed during the drive and was even able to fall asleep. The pain had again, *for the moment*, subsided.

The weekend was a continuation of pain off and on. There were periods of alleviation, but when it hit, I felt extremely miserable. I spent a lot of time in my massage chair, trying to get some relief. There were episodes when the pain was so strong, that it would wake me up in the middle of the night. I'd go to sit in the massage chair, trying to ease the suffering that I was feeling. I tried various things to try to get a reprieve from my misery. I was taking ibuprofen for the pain and I attempted using menthol and capsaicin creams on my back and neck. I tried pain patches, as well as a TENS unit. I even tried soaking in hot water baths with Epsom salts. *Nothing* helped! I was getting no relief.

I thought I would schedule a massage to see if it would bring a respite from the pain. I figured that I had a pinched nerve, perhaps a massage might help. The massage therapist that I called comes to your home for the massage. She came early Monday morning and gave me a great massage. There were parts of the massage that really hurt me, but I figured no pain, no gain. I went straight to bed after she left. I felt relaxed. However, by that afternoon the pain was back.

I decided that I had endured enough. I called my family doctor's office and made an appointment for the next morning. My usual doctor was not available, but I had an appointment with his colleague. I had seen him many times before, so this was acceptable to me. I also called and made an appointment for my younger daughter, remembering the episode at the water park when she fainted. She seemed to be feeling okay, but it still bothered me that I didn't know what had caused her to faint. I had told one of my friends (her husband is a heart patient) about what had happened. She suggested my daughter see a cardiologist just to rule out that this was not a heart related issue. I felt like it was a reasonable place to start and I knew it was better to be safe than sorry. I called and made her an appointment with the cardiologist we had met with the night of the ABI screening, Dr. Anil. He seemed to be very nice; someone that we could feel comfortable with. Her appointment was scheduled for Thursday, August 18, 2011.

Tuesday Morning, August 9, 2011

Once in the doctor's exam room, I related to him that I had been in a lot of pain for the past week. I told him I thought it must be a pinched nerve. The doctor agreed that was most likely the problem.

I have a friend who is a nurse. After my heart attack, I related this story to her. She told me to *NEVER* go into a doctor's office and offer my own diagnosis. She said to tell the doctor all your symptoms, but don't make your own assumption of what *you* think is wrong. If you do, the doctor may not think past your presumed diagnosis. This might bias the doctor from looking for the *real* cause of the problem. She said that many people make this mistake and compromise an accurate, unbiased assessment. I had never thought of this, but she was right. I guess that was exactly what I did that day.

The doctor prescribed anti-inflammatory medication, muscle relaxers, and pain pills. I have never been a person who liked to take a lot of medication; also I particularly didn't feel comfortable taking prescription pain pills. I have always felt that caution should be used when taking those types of medications, that they should be reserved for something more serious than just a pinched nerve. So, I had the anti-inflammatory and muscle relaxers filled, but told the pharmacist to hold the script for the pain pills. (I would be willing to bet they don't have customers make that request very often.) Even though I was in serious pain, I decided I would continue taking the ibuprofen.

I had an appointment scheduled that afternoon with the dentist. I had broken a filling and had planned to have it fixed that day. It seemed to take longer than I expected and my jaw really hurt. I do remember telling the dentist that I had been having some problems with my neck and back. His chair had a nice head support and as he worked on my tooth, he had angled the chair back with my feet elevated. I told him being in his dental chair had made my neck feel better than it had all day.

I started taking the anti-inflammatory medication. I was to take the muscle relaxer at bedtime. I could hardly wait until bedtime came to take it, and I hoped to wake up feeling better. The next morning, Wednesday, August 10, there was still no relief. I was getting exceedingly discouraged, so I called the massage therapist and she came out again. The massage felt good while it lasted. The problem was that the pain would shortly return.

The next day, Thursday, August 11, was my older daughter's wedding anniversary. I did *not* feel like celebrating. I remember the pain being so vehement that afternoon that I curled up on the sofa in the fetal position and just sobbed. I was in absolute agony! I called my younger daughter at work and asked her to go by the pharmacy on her way home. I decided to go ahead and have the pain pills filled. She brought them home, but they didn't help much. I was getting little relief. That fact should have been a clue that there was something serious going on inside me. I knew I needed to go back to see my family doctor.

CHAPTER 4

Friday, August 12, 2011

I awoke feeling no better than the day before. I could hardly stand the pain. I was able to get an appointment with my doctor for that afternoon. I didn't want to face the weekend feeling like this. My younger daughter drove me to the doctor's office for my appointment.

When I walked in, the receptionist took one look at me and said, "Ms. Kim you don't look so good."

I told her that I felt horrible and she insisted that I come straight to the back. I really must have looked bad, because that had *never* happened before. I went into the exam room to wait for the doctor. It was a short wait.

When he came in, I related *everything* about how I had been feeling. I explained that the pain was worse in my left shoulder blade. It would travel up into my neck and head. There was extreme, concentrated tightness across my body from shoulder to shoulder in front and in back, just below my neck. My left arm would ache at the top and go numb at the bottom. When I had shoulder surgery two years earlier, a screw was placed in the bone. I asked him if he thought that perhaps the screw was backing out. I wondered if that might be the cause of the pain and numbness, but he told me he didn't think so.

I then told him I had a piercing ache in my jaw. It was deep within the bone on the left edge on my jaw and felt similar to a toothache. It ached in an area of about a one inch width from the hinge of my jaw to just past my chin on the right side. I let him know I had been to the dentist three days earlier, and perhaps the fact that I had to keep my jaw open for an extended time might be contributing to my pain. The pain from my jaw would sometimes even radiate up into my left ear.

All these pains varied in intensity. At this point though, it would come and go in the sense that it would occasionally slack off in strength, though the pain would never go away completely. However, the severity was increasing and lasting for longer intervals.

As I am writing this in the present, I notice something that I didn't expect. As these unpleasant memories come flooding back, my chest and back are again feeling tight. I remember the pain vividly and actually feel anxious and uneasy. I'm breathing harder as I try to put all that I was feeling at that time on paper. It's most distressing because even the recollection of the pain is making me relive those horrific moments.

I have tried to be as specific with the details as I possibly could. My hope is, if anyone reading this has similar symptoms, you'll recognize these symptoms as being heart related, even though I did not. I would like to expound on another facet of the pain. At the time, I didn't really consider that this pain differed from pain that I'd felt before. When I think back now, I realize the pain was a squeezing or constricting type of pain. I know now that this was a key factor.

Let us go back to my doctor's visit. I know doctors hear complaints all day long, which must be the down side of their job. I would imagine they even become accustomed to hearing people routinely complain given that many of those complaints are just for minor things. That day though, I wanted my doctor to realize the way I was feeling was out of the ordinary for *me*. I only saw him a couple of times a year, but I reminded him that I had been coming to see him for about twenty-five years and he had *never* seen me come twice in the same week. "I'm no wimp, but this is really kicking my butt," I told him. I revealed to him that the pain was so intense that I would compare it to labor pains. I said on a scale of one to ten, I was sure this was *at least* a nine and a half. He agreed with his colleague's diagnosis of a pinched nerve. He told me to continue taking the medications, but he was going to increase the muscle relaxers. He wanted me to take it three times a day, instead of once at bedtime.

He was kind and appeared to listen to me. I think though, he was distracted that day. The reason I say this, is during my brief office visit, the nurse called him out of the exam room twice. The first time I could hear him in the hallway, on the phone with a patient. I was able to hear only one side of the conversation, but from what the doctor said, it sounded to me as if the person on the other end of the phone had an aortic aneurism. By what the doctor was telling that person, it seemed as if the person did not understand how vital it was to be treated promptly. The doctor was trying to stress the necessity of seeking speedy treatment. He hung up the phone and returned to the exam room. A minute or two later the nurse interrupted again. This time there was a phone call from another doctor. He left again and talked briefly to the other doctor. I was not able to discern if there was a relation between the two calls or not.

I honestly don't feel that he purposely ignored me. I know the health issues of that other person were serious and perhaps life threatening. He most likely had this serious matter weighing on his mind. Nevertheless, the interruptions I feel, distracted my doctor. Perhaps his focus was not on what I was saying. Perchance, these events may have affected how he perceived what I was telling him. For this reason, doctors should consider making a rule not to allow interruptions of their patient's visits, so that their concentration will not be broken.

There is one other interesting fact, as I think back. On that day and on my visit three days earlier my blood pressure was on the low side of normal. I would have expected it to be higher when you were having symptoms that would indicate the possible threat of a heart attack looming, but it was good just as it normally was. My visit was over; I gathered my script and paid my bill. I walked to the car and I was literally in tears. I felt *so* discouraged. I felt no better or hopeful than when I had walked in. I *just* wanted to *stop* hurting. All that I could contemplate was what was in store for me for the weekend. I feared a weekend of feeling miserable and in pain, and I wasn't looking forward to it.

I got into the car with my daughter and expressed how utterly distressed and discouraged I felt. She asked me what I wanted to do, and I told her that I couldn't face the weekend feeling like this. I needed to find some respite from the pain. I told her to drive me to the chiropractor's office in hopes that he could give me some sorely needed relief. That was our next stop.

I remember being in the treatment room lying face down on the table waiting for the chiropractor to come in. He walked in, offered a greeting, and proceeded to adjust my back. He didn't even ask about my problem. I remember feeling irritated with him because his approach appeared so rote and perfunctory.

I sat up, faced him and said, "Before you start, let me tell you what's going on with me."

I guess I was somewhat curt, because he later told me that I was very different that day. Think about it though, even a good old family pet will bite when they are hurting or injured. Thinking back in hindsight, I realize that he wasn't being unfeeling or uncaring, it was most likely just an oversight at the end of a long day. I went through the whole nine yards of symptoms just as I had done an hour or so earlier with my family doctor. I didn't leave anything out. He then adjusted my back and neck. I got some relief while he was working on me. However, by the time I got to my car, I was hurting again. *Oh, how was I going to get through this weekend?* I desperately needed to stop hurting! I had my muscle relaxers filled and went home. I went to bed and tried to rest.

The next day was Saturday; it wasn't much different from the previous day. The only difference was that I was sleeping more due to the increase in muscle relaxers. The next day, Sunday, August 14, was *dreadful*. I was in complete agony! I tried to reach the massage therapist, but was unsuccessful. I knew a few other people who did massages and tried to contact them. I was like an addict trying to score a fix. I was trembling in pain! No one was available on a Sunday afternoon. I planned to go *back* to the doctor's office the next morning. The pain was so excruciating that it was making me feel crazy. In the past, I've had a high tolerance to pain. That should have clued me in on the fact that this time, something was *very* different.

I know that you are perhaps wondering why I didn't go to the emergency room if I was in *that* much pain. I'll try to explain, but it is important to realize that I come from a long line of strong Cajun women. We are somewhat Spartan-like. Please don't interpret that to mean unfeminine, that is definitely not the case. We just come from strong, resilient stock. We are not wimpy, whiny, pampered women, and we don't want to be. We take charge and push through the pain. We certainly don't go to the emergency room for every little thing. There needs to be a limb dangling, intestines spilling out, or bleeding from the eyeballs in order to warrant a visit to the emergency room. My point being ... it has to be pretty serious in order for us to feel like we need to go. Although my pain *was* extremely intense, I thought it was simply back and neck pain. I figured there was little else they could do at the emergency room. They could give me drugs, but I was already taking those.

I had no idea that it could actually be my heart. If I had, I would have gone to see a cardiologist. I don't have any qualms about going to the doctor if there is a real need. I try to take an active role in my health and believe in preventative care. I've tried to be a good student of my own health. After all, who knows me better than me? In spite of this fact, I guess I missed the boat in this case.

That night, we went to bed earlier than usual. My husband had a big inventory audit at work that started the next morning. This annual three-day event was something, he was seriously dreading. He had been trying to get everything organized for it. We went to bed early so that he would feel rested for the big day ahead. This was going to be the worst three days at work out of the entire year. He is the most honest, hardworking, conscientious person that I know, always giving his best in all that he does. He wanted everything to turn out perfectly and I hoped for his sake that it would.

CHAPTER 5

Sunday Night, August 14, 2011

I took my pain pills, muscle relaxers, and *finally* drifted off to sleep ... The next thing I remember was being awakened out of a deep sleep, by the ringing of the phone. When it rang, I remember jumping, as if I was startled. It was about 8:00 a.m., Monday, August 15. My next-door neighbor was calling. It was not for any specific reason, "just to talk." This was completely out of character for her. She is usually a late sleeper and never calls this early. I didn't feel very talkative and remember telling her that I didn't feel well. I told her that I felt, "very out of it." We talked; well, mainly she talked for a little while. After I hung up the phone, I noticed something was different.

My shoulder blade for the first time in two weeks was not hurting or feeling tight. I thought that the pinched nerve had finally released and I was delighted. I thought maybe, just maybe, I would start to feel better now. I was relieved. After all this time I had suffered, perhaps this was the time to get better. I really did need that since I had been so utterly miserable.

I noticed though, that I felt bad physically. It's hard for me to be specific and describe *exactly* how I felt. I just felt bad; I had no energy, or strength, and seemed very lethargic. I felt totally drained and exhausted. I drug around, trying to compel myself to be active, but ended up in and out of bed all day. I forced myself to sit up on the sofa, but I still felt terrible. I didn't feel like eating either. By the afternoon, I began to notice that I had congestion in my chest. My younger daughter was off work that day and at about 3 p.m. I asked her to call the doctor's office to see if I could get in for an appointment. My intentions were to call for an appointment the first thing Monday morning. Conversely, when I awoke and the pain in my shoulder was gone, I assumed that I was on the upswing. I *could not* have been more wrong! My daughter called the doctor's office several times, but each time she called, she got a busy signal. It was getting closer to 5 p.m. so I told her to give up trying.

I talked with my mother on the phone and told her I was still feeling bad. She encouraged me to make an appointment with my doctor for Tuesday morning and she would drive me. I agreed and said I would call for an appointment as soon as the doctor's office opened.

I kept thinking about the congestion in my chest. I have several medical books written for the non-professional. I got them out and started searching. I came to the conclusion that I might be coming down with pneumonia. I had heard that this could be possible if a person was very inactive and I had been in the last two weeks. That coupled with the fact that I had been taking so many pain pills and muscle relaxers, made me feel like it could be feasible. I read all the symptoms and I had most of them, except for fever. I was going to the doctor's office first thing in the morning. So I felt like I would be all right until morning, even if it were pneumonia. I knew that pneumonia was serious, but not as serious as it used to be in times past.

I picked at my dinner and even though I didn't feel like it, I watched television with my family for a while. I just thought that sitting upright might make me feel better, since my chest felt deeply congested. I felt incredibly tired and decided to take a nap in my bedroom. I remember lying there in the dark, feeling very strange. I felt the congestion in my chest was worse than it had been earlier that day. In addition, I noticed an odd sound when I exhaled. It was a strange, long, high-pitched wheezing sound at the end of my exhalation and was completely involuntary. I had never experienced that before. I felt something different *inside* as well. Deep inside me, I had a feeling of dread. I was afraid to go to sleep. I feared not waking up. I had never felt like that before either. I remember praying. Praying—asking God to help me shake that awful feeling. I think that I *may* have nodded off to sleep for just a moment, but I was restless and anxious, so much so, that I got up and went back with my husband and daughter.

I did consider going to the emergency room, but I figured I would be all right until morning. I didn't want to go to the emergency room and run up a hospital bill if it wasn't really necessary. Besides that, what if it wasn't anything serious? I would have *felt silly*; I didn't want that either. I did tell my husband my suspicions—that I thought I may be coming down with pneumonia. He was concerned about me, but I decided to try to downplay how I was *really* feeling. I just couldn't let on that I felt as bad as I did. I knew that he was under a lot of pressure at work with his inventory. Everything had gone well that first day, one day down and two to go. We wanted to turn in early again so that he could get a good night's rest.

When we went to bed, I *couldn't* get comfortable. I noticed that my breathing was somewhat shallow. In an effort to try to get to sleep, I propped up with extra pillows and tried rubbing my chest with menthol rub. I knew that I must be disturbing my husband because of my twisting and turning. I began to realize that something was seriously wrong. I could feel a weight on my chest just below where my neck and chest met. I knew at that point that I probably should go to the hospital, but I really was hoping it would improve. It did not!

I should have told my husband earlier, but I think I was most likely trying to convince myself that this was *not* really happening. I guess partly, it was that strong Cajun woman thing still driving me. I feared that I was about to lose control over my life, *and I was*. I just had no idea to what extent at this point. I knew that my husband had such a stressful day ahead of him and I didn't want to add to his stress. This could not be happening at a worse time. I was trying to hide the fact that I was having difficulty breathing from my husband. My breathing was getting more and more shallow. I was getting panicky. I had never had to struggle for breath before. It's such an awful feeling as you fear that each breath could be your last. I knew that I couldn't wait any longer. It was near midnight when I sat up on the side of the bed. I awoke my husband when I did so because he asked me if I was going on the sofa in order to try to get more comfortable.

"No," I said, "I think I need to go to the hospital."

He turned on the lamp and looked at me in surprise and disbelief. He immediately jumped out of bed and started to get dressed. I changed clothes too, and grabbed my purse.

I went into my daughter's room to tell her where we were going. She had taken sinus medication before going to bed. She was evidently in a deep sleep ... and very incoherent. I tried again to wake her up, but it was not happening. We decided that we would call her later. I remember looking around my house as we were leaving. I had a very eerie feeling. I wondered if I would come back to it.

We walked out the door and my husband locked it.

"Wait! Unlock it," I told him, "I need to get something."

"What do you need?"

"I want to get an aspirin."

In a guarded tone paired with a strange look on his face, he said, "*Why?*"

"In case I'm having a heart attack." I said with precaution.

It had finally sunk in that it *could* be my heart. *Had I been in denial the whole time?* He sighed deeply and looked unnerved. That statement had shocked him, because he had been thinking that my issues were pneumonia related, as I had told him earlier. I went back into the house to get my aspirin and we then got into the car. My neck was hurting. I had my neck pillow in the car that I had used the day we went to the water park. I put it on, trying to increase my comfort on the ride to the hospital.

I had grabbed a handful of cough drops as well before leaving the house. I popped one into my mouth, with the hope it would help with my breathing. We drove for about four to five minutes in complete silence. My mind was racing. The silence between us told me that my husband's was too, as both of us were trying to sort out everything that was running through our heads. I think we were sensing in these moments that our lives were about to change. I then started to tell my husband things I wanted him to help me remember when we got to the emergency room. He was beginning to realize that this could be serious. He is a very nervous person and I could tell that he was becoming progressively more rattled.

I suggested that I call my sister to have her meet us at the emergency room. In my mind, this was more for him, for moral support, than for me. He agreed that would be a good idea. I called my sister's house and apologized for calling so late. I hated to wake her up because she had just come back from a trip the night before. I briefly explained what was going on. She said she would meet us at the emergency room.

We passed my parents home on the way to the hospital. I remember tearing up as we did so. I didn't want to call and worry them. I wanted to wait until we knew what was actually taking place. I was trying to hold it together, but it wasn't easy because I feared the worst. If this was indeed the worst, if this was indeed something serious, how were they going to handle this news?

CHAPTER 6

We arrived at the emergency room, but couldn't pull up because a car belonging to a pizza delivery person blocked the ramp. I guess someone needed a late night snack. I thought that my husband was going to *explode*! I would have hated to know what *his* blood pressure was at the time. He finally maneuvered around the pizza delivery car and pulled up to the emergency room doors.

I told him to let me out while he parked the car. He didn't want to leave me, but I assured him that I would be okay. The receptionist was just inside the doors. I walked in and the waiting room was *completely* empty. That was a first, and I was thankful. I sat down at the reception desk and started to give her my information. My husband was at my side before we were finished.

The receptionist ushered us to the back right away, to triage. The triage nurse had me put on a *lovely* hospital gown. She then took my blood pressure. It was low. I thought that was a good thing, however; I would shortly find out differently. She took my temperature, which was normal. Next, she did an EKG. She proceeded to ask me a series of questions. She asked about my symptoms. They were, first, shortness of breath. I felt like I had a weight on my chest. My neck hurt and I was congested. She took a brief history. I told her about the pain in my shoulder blade and neck for the past two weeks. I said that I wasn't sure if the two were related. I told her the pain that I had been experiencing was gone when I awoke that morning. She next asked about the medications I was taking. I dreaded telling her about the pain pills and muscle relaxers. I was concerned she may think I was one of those people who take these types of medications on a regular basis. I knew that some who abused drugs, will go to the emergency room in an effort to get more drugs. I didn't want the hospital staff to think that of me. My sister had arrived by this time and they had allowed her to come back to triage with us.

The nurse then told us that we could all follow her. I reached for the airy gap of my lovely open-backed gown and followed her to one of the exam rooms down the hall. I felt a bit encouraged. I figured that my EKG must have looked fairly good since they were letting me walk to the back, instead of putting me in a wheel chair. I thought, perhaps I wasn't having a heart attack after all. Maybe I had come for nothing. Had I possibly overreacted? I was actually not sure what I should think at this point.

The nurse got me settled in the exam room and the emergency room doctor came in shortly. He asked some of the same questions that the nurse had just asked. I went through them again. I told him I wondered if perhaps I had pneumonia. There I was *again* giving my own diagnosis. He checked me over and listened to my heart and lungs. He next ordered blood work, a chest X-ray and a breathing treatment. They brought in a portable X-ray machine and shot pictures of my lungs.

A friendly man from respiratory therapy came in to do a breathing treatment for me. They then placed an oxygen cannula in my nose to help my breathing. I was at that moment thinking that maybe I was right; maybe it was pneumonia after all. A little later, I received a second breathing treatment. It was helping a little bit, I was breathing a little easier and I was finally more comfortable. I even joked with the respiratory therapist about the breathing treatment. I told him I felt like I was smoking. That was a first for me, because I had never smoked in my life. He told me that was a good thing, since smoking was so bad for your health. The mood seemed lighter and I noticed that my husband didn't seem as tense. I too, was feeling more relaxed but, shortly that atmosphere would drastically change.

The door to the exam room opened and the emergency room doctor walked in again.

He looked at me and bluntly said, "You've had a heart attack, you've been having angina pains, you're in heart failure, and we're admitting you."

I was totally and completely stunned. With eyes wide from disbelief I responded, "You've *got* to be kidding!"

He retorted, "No, I'm not kidding."

My next question was, "When?"

He said, "I can't say exactly when, but *at least* eight hours prior to your coming in."

We would later surmise that the event occurred sometime prior to my waking up on Monday morning. It was now the early hours of Tuesday, August 16. At least eighteen hours (perhaps more) had gone by since that time. This was some time before my neighbor called me on Monday morning. When I think about it now, I wonder, did she inadvertently save my life? If she had not called me that morning, what would have happened? Would I have just continued to sleep? Would my heart just have gotten weaker and weaker? Did the ringing of the phone startle me and get my heart pumping? Would I have just died in my sleep? I will never know the actual answers to these questions. It does give one something to ponder though. Months later, I read an article that chilled me. It stated that 60% of people who had a heart attack in their sleep—*did not* wake up.

I had just found out I had a heart attack and that I was in heart failure. Thinking back, I'm still astounded by the frankness of the emergency room doctor. Why couldn't he break it to me gently? I mean ... I had *just* had a heart attack ... was he trying to give me another one? This was the craziest moment of my life! I was in shock and utter disbelief! I am pretty sure that my husband and sister were too.

"But I *wanted* it to be pneumonia," I idealistically admitted to the doctor.

With a half-smile and a shake of his head, he looked at me and said, "Well you don't get a choice." And ... he was right.

The next moments were like a whirlwind. It was as if I were on a carnival ride that was spinning unrestrained. In the blink of an eye, things had accelerated into hyperdrive. My life was upside down and wobbling erratically out of control. As if to add to the frenzy, the emergency room staff went into rapid action like an episode of *E.R.* But *this time* ... *I* would be the patient. As much as I loved that show, with its riveting, fast-paced, medical drama, I did *not* want to be the star of this insane episode.

The moments that followed were surreal; I remember them clearly. I was lying on the exam room table, but it was as if I were watching this whole drama unfold from the sidelines. I seemed to be an observer, as well as the patient. There was a flurry of activity in the room. There was a nurse starting an I.V. on my right. On my left was another giving me injections. I asked, what was their purpose? She told me that they were blood thinners. Upon hearing this, my already wounded heart felt like it sank. Injection number one, injection number two, the nurse said the next one had to be given in my stomach. I asked, "Why so many blood thinners?" The nurse explained that they all worked in different ways. She said I would need them because I was going to have heart catheterization, or an angiogram. The injection given in the stomach is administered with a thrust of force behind it, and it *hurts*! The area would stay sore and bruised for weeks. This was the first of its kind, but not the last. They next affixed leads to my chest to monitor my heartbeat. My oxygen levels and blood pressure were being monitored as well. In addition, I was given an assortment of medications orally.

There is another injection. Again, I asked what was its purpose? The nurse said that it was a diuretic, and a large dose. This was to help me to void fluid. There was a considerable build up of fluid in my lungs. That was why I was having shortness of breath. The nurse told me that I would need to be able to lie flat on my back for the heart catheterization procedure. It was necessary first to void the fluid that had built up in my lungs in order to accomplish this. All this activity was in order to prep me to go to the Cardiac Care Unit (CCU), until the fluid issue was resolved. Then, they would perform the angiogram. This procedure uses X-ray imaging to determine if there are blockages in your coronary arteries. During the angiogram, a contrast-type dye that is visible by X-ray is used. As the dye is injected, the X-ray machine takes a series of images. Using this method, they are able to determine if there are any blockages present and how well the heart muscle is functioning. This also provides a detailed look at the blood flow to the arteries of the heart.

The idea that there was a *possibility* that open-heart surgery *may* be necessary was introduced at this time. That outcome would depend on what was revealed during the angiogram. I felt very frightened and felt that this *must* be a bad dream, that none of this could possibly be real. In a small, fearful voice, I asked the nurse to my left, "What causes a heart attack?" I was like an innocent little child asking, "Why is the sky blue?" She rattled off several reasons why, none of which I can remember now, except one. She said that sometimes a blockage could occur in the coronary arteries that supply blood to the heart muscle. This blockage can then result in a heart attack.

I was listening to her, but thinking to myself, "A blockage? I don't think I have a blockage. I would probably feel this if I did." She concluded with, "Some people have heart attacks without any blockage." All I could think was, *"That's* got to be what's happening to me. It can't be a blockage because I'm only 55 years old. For the most part, I watch my diet. I don't smoke. I never have … So why did this happen?" It seemed that being told I might possibly have a blockage struck a nerve. I guess, I somewhat viewed it as an attack on my character. As if she were implying I didn't take care of my health when I knew that I had tried. I realize now that reaction was the stress of the moment. I guess learning that you're in heart failure can have that effect on you. It was a lot to absorb in a very short time.

Some of the activity was slowing down. They were telling me that I would shortly be taken to CCU. Once in CCU, my husband and sister would be allowed to visit for a little while, but would not be allowed to stay. CCU has a very strict visitation policy.

My husband, my sister and I were alone now, waiting for me to be transported to CCU. We were all still in shock. I *kept* repeating, "I can't believe this. This is unreal." I looked at my husband who was leaning against the wall to my right (probably so that he wouldn't fall over).

In a soft, sheepish voice I said, "I always thought that it would be you and not me." That rather broke the tension in the room.

He facetiously replied, "Gee, thanks."

With a sigh, I told him, "You know what I mean."

"I know what you mean; but this is why I've wanted you to take better care of yourself, instead of worrying so much about me," he firmly said.

He fully realized that I stressed more over *his* health, than my own. There was no way I could deny it because he was right.

CHAPTER 7

We now needed to shift gears. We had to start thinking ahead. As I said earlier, we had left our daughter (age 22) at home asleep. I didn't want her to wake up and wonder why her parents had simply vanished in the middle of the night. For that reason, my husband was going home to wake her up and fill her in on everything that had taken place while she was sleeping. She worked at the hospital where I was now a patient. She normally started her shift around 5:30 a.m.; therefore, she would be getting up just after 4:00 a.m. I wanted him home before she woke up. I gave him a list of things that I would need from home, so that he could bring them to me when he returned.

I apologized to him because I felt guilty about keeping him up all night, *especially* in the middle of his inventory. He reassuringly told me not to worry about that, just to concentrate on getting better. In addition, I told him that I wanted him to report for work when it was time because I felt doing so would keep his mind occupied instead of just worrying and waiting. He resolutely asserted that he just couldn't leave, but despite what he said I *insisted* because I knew how important this inventory was to him. His being there was essential to the project. He was responsible and accountable for parts and equipment worth millions of dollars. I reminded him that they were not going to allow him to stay in CCU with me anyway. I felt he would feel less worried if he would stay busy and keep his mind engaged. I assured him that someone would call before the angiogram so that he could come back. Lastly, I pleaded, "Pleeaassee?" and he *finally* agreed to go. He should have realized it is just *pointless* to argue with a woman on a gurney headed for CCU.

We next discussed the others who needed to be notified. There was our daughter who lives in New Orleans, my parents, and our closest friends. I didn't want anyone getting this disturbing phone call in the wee hours of the morning. I've always felt that for some reason bad news seemed so much worse when it's still dark, so I asked them to wait until sunrise to start calling people. They agreed. I still felt somewhat in charge of my life, still giving orders, but that was my only power at this point.

Next, I was transported via gurney, to CCU, my new home for the next three days. The nurse got me settled. Well, as settled as one could be, given recent events. She took my vitals and tried to make me more comfortable. She was soft-spoken, gentle and had a manner about her that reflected a compassionate, caring attitude. She let me know she was just outside if I needed anything and then said she would go to get my family to visit me for just a short while.

The way that CCU is set up; there is one nurse for every two patients with her desk in between the two rooms. The front of the patient's room is glass so that she can watch over the patient at all times and vital signs are on a computer screen in front of her. A patient can buzz her if there is a real need, but she is so close that she will hear you if you simply call out. That close proximity gave me a feeling of security. In addition, her sweet, kind demeanor was very comforting to me at such a crazy time in my life.

My family came back to see me and I added a few more things to my husband's list of things to bring back. I was anxious for him to go home before my daughter awoke, even though I really hated for him to leave me. I worried he might be distracted while driving home since I knew he now had a lot on his mind. I told him I loved him, but that's something I do every day. This time it felt more intense. I didn't want it to be the last time he would hear me say it. I begged him to be careful because I knew how stressed he was, not to mention that he hadn't slept that night.

He went home and my sister stayed. We discussed at length the events of the past couple hours. I was having a hard time wrapping my mind around the idea that I had a heart attack, was in heart failure and *didn't* even realize it. I felt better with my sister there. She is my only sibling and we are nine and a half years apart. She enjoys telling people that I am the *older* sister.

I was thrilled when she was born. However, when she got old enough to dig in my room and my stuff, I didn't like her as much. As we got older though, the age gap between us narrowed and we became the same age—and friends. There's no sibling rivalry between us now. We aren't competitive with each other; I feel that competition has no place in families. In fact, I view it as very divisive and therefore destructive. My sister is an extremely talented person, and I'm proud of her success. Our family is certainly not the "Cleavers." We are not all huggy, huggy and kissy, kissy, but we are a close-knit family who loves fiercely and will stand beside each other no matter what. We know that we can depend on one another and have each other's back.

My sister has had her own share of trials. She lost her husband in a car accident at the age of 23. The day that her husband died their only child turned 11 months old. That was a very dark and difficult time in her life. Throughout this unfortunate event, she displayed strength and dignity. She got through those unhappy days and found a brighter future. She did remarry a very kind and upstanding man who is exceptionally good to her and to my niece.

I was glad that she was there because she reminded me of several things I needed to remember regarding my health care. I think it is always a good idea to have someone else with the patient, someone who will look out after the patient's best interests. Due to the stressful situation of an illness and the influence of drugs, patients *aren't* always their own best advocate.

We next discussed her going to tell our parents when morning came. We agreed that was a job best handled in person, not over the phone. My father is a very quiet, laid-back person. He is a good, generous, and hard-working man. My mother too, is good, generous, and hardworking. However, she is *extremely* nervous. She worries excessively, especially about her family. She has past issues that have certainly contributed to that.

At age 12, she was in a freak accident. She had gone to spend the night with her grandmother. Her grandmother's home was located at the end of a small peninsula that rested on the Atchafalaya River near Berwick, LA. The accident happened in the early morning hours, before daybreak. A tugboat captain pushing a line of barges fell asleep at the wheel. The barges ran aground, destroying her grandmother's old wooden house. My mother was asleep on the floor next to her grandmother's bed—a heavy iron bed. I am positive that the void next to the iron bed is what saved her life.

She was pinned within the wreckage, impaled with nails through her arms. She was trapped, unable to move. The kitchen, which was on the opposite end of the house, caught fire. Thankfully, workers that were onboard the boat, put it out quickly. They also heard my mother's cries for help and fortunately, she was safely pulled from the wreckage. Her uncle was also injured in the accident. Sadly, she would learn that her grandmother died from a blow to her temple when the house collapsed.

The trauma of these events, I feel must be the reason behind her feeling nervous and anxious much of the time. How could you experience something like this and remain unaffected? She said at that time, counseling was completely unheard of in the small town where she lived. I personally feel she must be affected by some type of post-traumatic stress even though there was never a professional diagnosis. My heart goes out to her for all of the anxiety that she deals with. She never lets it stop her though. Many, who know her, are not even aware of the trauma that she has experienced. The way that she has coped despite the odds is a testament to her strength and character. She is a root of that strong Cajun stock that I mentioned earlier. We sometimes joke that she has a lot in common with the Wicked Witch of the East in the Wizard of Oz. She had a house fall on her too.

We dread any serious news because we don't want to see her unduly stressed. My sister was the one elected to the job of telling her about me. My sister and I both tend to have a wry sense of humor and that aspect became apparent in her next statement.

My sister tells me, "Sure you've got the easy job. You get to lounge around here in CCU, I have to face Mama."

I needed that humorous break. We both laughed for the first time. My breathing is somewhat easier now. Between the breathing treatments, the oxygen, and the diuretics starting to kick in, I was getting some relief. I was not in any real pain. I was just uncomfortable.

CHAPTER 8

My husband came back and my daughter was with him. Since she worked there at the hospital, she was able to use her I.D. badge to come directly to CCU. Due to the fact that most of the patients are in serious condition, entry is regulated in CCU and there are strict visiting hours for this reason.

She walked in looking so scared and that's a look I'll never forget. The expression on her face looked as if she had been physically wounded. She anxiously expressed how worried she was. I told her that I was going to be okay, not to worry. I wasn't completely convinced of that myself, but I did just as any mother would do to comfort her child. Poor thing, when we had all gone to bed the night before, it was just a routine night like any other. However, the following morning wasn't routine at all. She awakened to her dad telling her that I was in the hospital, and that I had suffered a heart attack. It was hard for her to process what had taken place while she slept. I knew *exactly* how she felt.

I assured her that I was going to be all right. Her shift for work started in less than an hour and she told me she was going to report for work to explain that she couldn't stay and would then be back to stay with me. I told her that I was fine, to go ahead to work. I thought like my husband, her keeping busy would be the best thing for her. She protested, but I insisted. I told her since I was nearby, she could check on me frequently. I felt that staying busy would keep her mind occupied, giving her less time to stress and worry over me. I thought it would be better for her to wait to get off work when I had the angiogram scheduled for later that morning. She didn't want to comply, but I finally got her to reluctantly agree. She gave my nurse her extension number and told her to call with any change. I really hoped that staying busy would keep her mind off the seriousness of the situation.

The nurse had been very lenient with my visitors, but she told them they would now have to leave since she wanted me to try to get some rest. I told my husband to go to work and try to finish what he needed to do. The angiogram was scheduled for 11:00 a.m. and he was going to come back before that time.

I could see in their troubled faces that no one wanted to leave. I knew that it was very difficult for them and extremely hard for me too. All I could think of was, "Suppose something goes wrong before they get back." I worried if it did, they would blame themselves for not staying with me and I didn't want them to have *any* regrets or guilt to deal with. I also worried with so much on their minds they would become distracted or possibly careless. Still, I hoped that doing normal things would help them cope with this insane situation. I have to say, I was unsure if sending them away was the right decision.

I felt so torn. I *really* wanted them here close to me, to cling to for comfort and reassurance, but I was trying to do what was best for them too. I hoped that I had made the right decision—for *all* of us.

I was alone now ... alone with my thoughts. The room was dark and quiet. My mind was filled with dark thoughts, but *not* quiet in the least. My mind was racing, darting from one disquieting thought to another. I was trying to process a flood of questions, but I couldn't find *any* satisfying answers. I felt a torrent of mixed emotions that left me with an empty, aching feeling in the pit of my stomach as well. There was an internal monologue going on in my head that was interspersed with prayer. I *wanted*, and *needed* to talk to God, and I did. The problem was that my mind would continuously wander. It was as if someone was flipping through the channels on a television. I would then come back to my prayers. The following are some of my recollections of the jumbled thoughts that were whirling around in my head at that time.

I think that my first contemplation was, "*why?*" not, "why me?" I have come to understand, "why me?" is what most people ask. I knew in the Bible at Ecclesiastes 9:11 it tells us that time and unexpected events overtake us all. This surely was an unexpected event. I certainly didn't blame God as some people do when bad things happen. I knew that sometimes, bad things just happen to good people ... I understood that. This "*why?*" was, "Why did this happen in the first place? What could have caused this?" I was only 55 years old and I lived a good, wholesome lifestyle. I had never smoked, nor was I around second-hand smoke for any great lengths of time. I didn't drink, unless you call 3-4 drinks a *year*, drinking.

It simply wasn't something I really enjoyed, so I just didn't do it. I figured why waste the carbs anyway? I had never done illegal, or for that matter, legal drugs. Those are all risk factors, but they didn't apply to me. So, I needed to know, "*WHY?*"

In search of answers, I reviewed my medical history. I knew that high blood pressure was a major contributing factor to heart issues. However, I had never had high blood pressure. My blood pressure was usually on the low side of normal, so I could rule that out as a cause.

I did have Hypothyroidism and I had been taking medication to treat this condition for about fourteen years. A year earlier, I was diagnosed with Hashimoto's disease or Hashimoto's thyroiditis, which is an autoimmune disease of the thyroid. With this disorder, the body's natural defenses against infection react against the proteins in the thyroid gland, resulting in a gradual destruction of the gland, eventually rendering it unable to produce thyroid hormones. As far as I knew, these conditions were under control.

For as long as I was aware that I had a thyroid condition, I had noticed that my heartbeat was rapid. I also experienced heart palpations occasionally, and sometimes more frequently than occasionally. I had asked a doctor about this when it first started to occur. She told me that the thyroid issues caused it and it was normal with hypothyroidism. Since it was supposed to be normal, I tried to dismiss it. What I didn't know then, was that hypothyroidism can put a woman at greater risk for heart disease since hypothyroidism elevates blood cholesterol and triglycerides. It can also increase the risk for blood sugar disorders, which in turn, can cause insulin resistance.

I had started seeing an endocrinologist twenty months earlier; after I discovered I was pre-diabetic. When I became aware of this, I really did take it seriously and I felt that it was my wake-up call. Along with seeing an endocrinologist, I sought nutrition counseling and can honestly say, I took the counsel to heart. I read labels; I drastically cut back on carbs. I tried to incorporate as many complex carbs and high fiber foods as I could into my diet. I read up on diabetes and I learned about the role the liver plays in the production of glucose and that I should watch my fats more carefully. I was *really* trying.

Here in the heart of Cajun Country, we have a reputation for delicious Cajun Cuisine. In fact, we are famous for it. In our culture, we take our food very seriously as it is an important part of our lives. *Everything* that we do would seem to revolve around food. If someone dies, we bring food. When a new baby is born, we bring food. Food is the remedy of choice no matter what the problem or occasion. Even the success or failure of a wedding is gauged by the food choices and/or quantity. If you ask a Cajun, "How was the wedding?" You will usually hear one of two answers. "It was so nice, the food was so good." or "That wedding was a disaster, they ran out of food." Cajun people will quickly and proudly tell you that they *"live to eat,"* instead of eating to live.

Therefore, it's not surprising that in South Louisiana there is a prevalence of obesity and diabetes, which means that our area is also at greater risk for heart disease. Some say that our food is, "to die for," but that *does not* have to be literal. I'm a pretty good cook, so I looked for new ways to redo the foods that we enjoyed. In that way our meals could taste good and be good for us. I found ways to modify most of those recipes so that we could eat our traditional dishes without them being a hazard to our health. We ate out occasionally, but I found it easier to stick to my diet when I prepared it myself. I must have been doing something right; my HbA1C (a blood test that measures glucose levels over the preceding months) was good in the blood work done in the emergency room that night.

This was not the first time that I had made dietary changes. When my father had his first heart attack in 1993, it was my first wake-up call. At the time though, I didn't totally think *I* was at risk because *I* was a woman after all. I mainly made the changes back then for my husband's sake; I was concerned about *his* risk. At this point, I started specifically watching our fat intake more carefully since this was recommended by my father's cardiologist.

The endocrinologist had been very encouraging and told me if I watched my diet, took my medication, and lost weight, my pre-diabetes might not progress into full-blown diabetes. That was what I wanted, that was my goal because I knew diabetes was a very dangerous disease. Therefore, I knew it would require a concerted, disciplined effort on my part to fight against it. I didn't do it perfectly, but my eating habits had improved considerably. I had also stepped up my activity level. I had never had an abundance of energy, but I was no couch potato either. I felt at the time, I was fortunate to discover the problem before it had progressed and caused irreparable damage.

Over several months, I had lost ten pounds. I still had a long way to go, but I did feel better. Weight loss not only makes you feel better physically, it makes you feel better about yourself as well. I still needed to lose another twenty to twenty-five pounds but I was at least moving in the right direction. Weight loss has never come easy for me. I knew that the thyroid issues made it more difficult because the lack of thyroid hormone slows down the metabolism for the entire body. I felt that I was being pro-active about my health; at least I was trying to be. After the initial ten pounds, my weight loss came to a halt. I wasn't really sure why, I was still being very selective about my food choices.

The endocrinologist had also discovered through blood work that I had a vitamin D insufficiency. An insufficiency is not as severe as a deficiency, but it does require attention. I had been able to bring my levels up to normal ranges by taking supplemental vitamin D, on a daily basis. I would learn later that this vitamin D insufficiency might have played some part in my heart disease as well.

CHAPTER 9

In view of all these improvements, I was back to the question of, *"why?"* Besides the help from the endocrinologist and the nutritionist, I had my mentor's help. My mentor was Doctor Oz. I watched Doctor Oz as often as I could. Sometimes I watched twice a day, so as not to miss anything. I always watched with notebook and pen in hand, jotting down anything that I felt ever applied to my family, my friends or me.

Anyone who knows me, or spends *any* length of time around me, will hear the following: "Doctor Oz says this" or "Doctor Oz says that." My husband, like many other husbands out there, *rolls his eyes* when I say this. He even refers to him as my "boyfriend." My older daughter has heard me quote him so much that she sarcastically refers to him as "Doctor God." I glare at them and tell them not to make fun of Doctor Oz! What men fail to realize is that Doctor Oz is helping us, as women, take better care of ourselves. In turn, we can live longer to be able to take care of *them*. That is a win-win situation in my opinion.

Like so many women, I like and respect what he has to say. He shows that he genuinely cares and is concerned about people. The advice he gives is good, practical advice that is relatable to the way he is conservative in his recommendations. What I really appreciate about him most is that he seems so down to earth. He is like a dear old friend that we feel comfortable with and can trust. Because of this, we his viewers, feel like we know him personally. After all, we all invite him into our homes on a daily basis. The other quality that resonates with so many women is that he is a devoted husband and father. Mrs. Oz must not be a jealous woman, not that such a beautiful woman need be. It is just that it must be so bizarre having all those women continually fawn over your husband, everywhere he goes.

I had learned *a lot* since I started watching his show. I *had* been applying *many* of the things that I was learning. So, I am thinking, "How could *I* have had a heart attack? I watch *Doctor Oz*!" I had been listening to what he was saying. Did I miss the episode on the warning signs? I didn't think I had.

The part that blew my mind was how could I have had a heart attack and not realized it? Or, as a typical Cajun would colloquially say, "How could I have *'caught'* a heart attack and not realized it?" How could I have not interpreted the symptoms and put the pieces together? I had been suffering for two weeks. How could I have missed that? If the emergency room doctor had said, "You are *having* a heart attack," I would have accepted that better than, "You *had* a heart attack."

I described my symptoms in detail some pages back. Everyone thinks about one symptom, when you think of a heart attack and that symptom was missing in my case. It was chest pain. I didn't experience chest pain, no, not even *once*. Don't get me wrong, I certainly don't feel like I missed out on something, it's just that's what we all expect to happen. I am totally confident that if my pain had been in my chest, I would have gone to see a cardiologist. I've since read that 40% of women that have heart attacks have no chest pain at all.

So, how was I to know it was my heart? Even my family doctor hadn't interpreted my symptoms as being heart related. I had seen a cardiologist four years earlier. At the time, I reasoned I was in my fifties now; I had reached that "over the hill mark." I figured it wouldn't hurt to have my heart checked out. They performed an EKG and a stress test and everything checked out fine at that time. I just never went back. *A lot* had evidently changed in four years.

I guess part of it boils down to denial too. It was as if not going back to hear there was a problem, then no problem existed. Sometimes many of us are afraid to know the truth. In our minds we think, if we don't hear it from a professional source, then it's not a reality. This, I believe, is called the "ostrich syndrome." I've heard many people say, "I don't want to know if I have something really bad." In some cases, ignorance can be bliss, but this *doesn't* apply where serious health issues are involved. To "know," means that you can do something about it, at least you have the *possibility* of changing your future for the better. Sadly, another reason that many often neglect their health is because they don't want to be labeled by having their health issues documented by a professional source. They are afraid that somewhere down the road, insurance companies or others will use this information against them as a "pre-existing condition."

In my quest for answers, I thought about the fact that my cholesterol was high and I wondered if that had played a part. I had heard so many people complain about the side effects of cholesterol medicine and sincerely felt that it might do more harm than good. I had heard it said that the medical community kept changing the guidelines for what is considered healthy levels. It used to be that they didn't want your cholesterol over 300. Now they were saying that it should be below 200. You hear all sorts of ideas, *especially* while waiting in the doctor's office. I would hear people say that they thought that this "cholesterol medicine thing" was a scheme cooked up between the doctors and the pharmaceutical companies just to make money, and I had even read a newspaper article to that effect. It was as if there was this whole conspiracy theory going on, I guess I halfway believed it too. I had also heard many people complain about muscle pain and cramps in their legs and I didn't want that either.

There was another reason that I had refused to take it. I had a very *personal* reason. My mother-in-law had passed away in December of 1999. At the start of that year, she was diagnosed with high cholesterol, but she appeared to be in good health otherwise. Her doctor had put her on a popular brand of cholesterol medication, not even attempting to try diet changes first.

After she was on the medication for a short while, she showed signs of elevated glucose levels in her blood work. Her doctor concluded that she was diabetic and then prescribed a diabetes medication for her. There are many diabetes medications on the market from which to choose. As a drug of *first choice*, the FDA did not recommend the medication that her doctor chose to prescribe. The recommendation for this particular medication was for more serious, advanced cases. Damage progressed quickly, despite her taking it for only for a short while. The FDA later recalled this same medication because of the indication of serious liver problems. There was clinical evidence that severe liver damage could occur, even after short-term use. My mother-in-law had liver cancer that progressed very quickly, resulting in her death.

We wanted answers. After her death, we did research and found out that the cholesterol medication she was taking can cause an elevation of blood glucose levels. It's not common, but it does happen. Before taking the cholesterol medication she didn't appear to be diabetic, in fact, she had blood work done right before starting the cholesterol medication. We concluded that the cholesterol medication had caused a false positive for diabetes.

We strongly felt that the cholesterol medication had been the first link in a chain of events that culminated in her death. We knew that use of the cholesterol medication had not *directly* caused her death. However, we did have very strong reservations against it because of the role that it played. These facts were the driving, negative factors that influenced my decision not to take these types of medications.

I next thought about my father. He was sixty-two when he had his first heart attack. He was sixty-nine when he had his second one. Was this my reason? Was it genetics? When he had his first heart attack, he had blockages that were opened and stented. A stent is a metal, wire-mesh tube that is put in place to keep a coronary artery open during the process of angioplasty. The stent stays in the artery permanently and the artery wall eventually covers the wire-mesh tube, as it grows around it.

When my father's stents were put in place, they were still in the clinical trial stage and were not approved for general use until more than a year later. At the time, the cardiologist explained the details about the stent to us, and asked for my mother's permission to use them. My father was in the process of having the heart attack at the time, so he could not give consent himself. After the fact, my father signed paperwork giving permission for them to be used. At that time, we had not even heard of a stent, but we know now that they saved his life that day.

Before stents were available, balloon angioplasty was performed to open blocked coronary arteries. However, this treatment was not always successful in the long term, because arteries can reclose without the stent to keep it open. There is less chance of this occurring with a stent in place. Little did my father know at that time, he was pioneering the way for his own daughter, eighteen years down the road.

He did well for a while, but seven years later, he had the second heart attack. This time open-heart surgery was required; the result was a triple bypass. I remember seeing him awake for the first time after surgery the next morning in CCU. He was holding his red heart pillow against his chest. He told us he felt like he had been run over by a truck. He was in so much pain. Was that going to happen to me? Was I facing surgery? I desperately hoped the answer was no.

Besides the pain of surgery, I had a fear of being anesthetized. Years earlier, I had gone to school with a young man who underwent a simple wrist operation. He was healthy and in his early twenties *but* he never woke up. After that, being put to sleep was a concern of mine because I realized that anesthesia carried certain risks. Even though that was a concern, it paled in comparison to the idea of open-heart surgery. I knew how serious that was. The nurse had introduced the idea of that possibility to me in the emergency room. The angiogram would be the deciding factor as to whether surgery would be necessary.

There was another thing that came to my mind. I had serious problems several years back with varicose veins in my legs and had several different types of treatments done to correct the problem. I had EVLT, which is laser ablation of the veins, a procedure that heats up the lining of the vein causing it to shut down. I had four or five phlebectomies to remove some of the affected veins. I also had sclerotherapy; this is when the vein is injected with an irritant that causes the vein to scar internally and eventually shut down. I knew that when certain veins in the legs are shut down, other dormant veins take over to compensate. I couldn't help but wonder though if I did need bypass surgery, were there any suitable, useable veins remaining that could be harvested? I would later learn when there are no suitable veins in the legs, a mammary artery in the chest can be used for this purpose.

I was told in the emergency room that I was in heart failure. That sounds *exceedingly* scary to hear. It's as if this eminent death sentence has just been issued, when in fact, that isn't necessarily the case. This condition, also known as congestive heart failure, occurs when the weakened heart pumps blood out with less force than is required. When blood returns to the heart faster than it can be pumped out, it gets backed up or is congested. This no doubt, was what was causing the fluid to collect in my lungs, making me short of breath.

My paternal grandmother died as a result of heart failure. This was the consequence of having type-1 diabetes for forty plus years. Back at the time when she was diagnosed, she didn't have the treatment options and resources that are available today and this took a tremendous toll on her heart. I didn't want that to be my fate.

Just hearing a doctor say "You're in heart failure" is so fear provoking and upsetting. When we think about our bodies, most of our body parts come in pairs, we have built-in spares. Even the vital organs that are singular, when they stop working there is a time delay before our death results. *Not so with our heart!* We only get one and when it stops, our life is over. *But I didn't want it to be over.* I had my wonderful family that depended on me, and I *needed* and *wanted* to be there for them.

CHAPTER 10

"What about my family?" My thoughts shifted away from me ... to *them*. "What would they do if I didn't survive? How would they manage without me?" I thought about my wonderful husband—my best friend and soul mate. He is good, kind, and supportive and for almost thirty-nine years of marriage, we have had a loving and faithful relationship. In fact, I feel like my *real life* started the day that we were married. We're the ideal match because we balance one another due to our different strengths and weaknesses. We have always done our best to take care of each other. I take care of running the house and paying the bills, in general taking care of *any* family business that arises. I think that's probably what most wives do. My husband couldn't tell you what bill is due, or for how much if his very life depended on it. That was my job. I thought, "If I don't make it, how's he going to survive?" The loss would put such a load on him. I remember how his dad grieved after his mom died. He found it so difficult to cope because he depended on her so much. I didn't want that for my husband, I didn't want to leave him. We married very young and have been truly devoted to one another over the years. We have so much in common and still enjoy each other's company, even after all these years. We may not be perfect, but we are the perfect match for one another. We would be so lost without each other.

I next thought about my two beautiful daughters, both grown now. I remember as a young mother, I always hoped that I would be able to finish raising them myself. I had a friend who was killed in a car accident, years ago and she left behind a seven-year-old daughter. While her husband eventually remarried someone very nice, it was still a loss for mother *and* daughter. They both were cheated because they had missed out on each other's lives. I didn't want that. I wanted to be able to raise my girls *myself*, and I felt blessed to be able to do so. They were now ages thirty-one and twenty-three and I was truly grateful for being a part of their lives for this long... *but it was not enough.*

You might reason, they're older, they don't need me now, but you would be *wrong*! I still needed my mother even though I was fifty-five. My mother had lost her mother nearly three years earlier at age ninety-eight and she wasn't ready even then. When you have a good, loving parent, you want them to be around forever. A mom is supposed to be there to love, to help, to guide, to be the family historian, to comfort, or just to listen. *That* is what a mother does. These children, these gifts from God, they are an *extension* of ourselves and we *need* one another. I knew that my girls still needed me to be a part of their lives, and I wanted so desperately to be there. I hoped and prayed that I would see the next day and their beautiful, sweet faces.

My parents needed me there too. I thought, "This is crazy, they are getting older now. They're at a point in their lives when they need me more now than ever to help them." How was I going to be able to do that? What condition was I in now? I couldn't die; I still had so many things I wanted to accomplish. I still had *so* much to do, but I was aware that death does not show respect for our personal agendas.

Some years back, I remember going to the visitation for the father of a friend. Several people in attendance were discussing death and giving their different viewpoints on the subject. I recall one person saying they feared the thought of being dead; the thought of being "non-existent" was a serious concern to them. I remember saying, "I don't fear *being* dead. I fear the dying process, getting from point A to point B." In light of recent events I reasoned, "Was I possibly facing that prospect, maybe even today?" I decided that I had changed my mind! I knew with certainty in those moments that God had put eternity into my heart and I was not ready to give that up. I knew if I passed away under sedation, the dying process would be as easy as it gets. I have heard this kind of death called the "easy death" or "the good death," but I wanted to *live*! I did not want to be "*non-existent*," I wanted to be here with my family and friends. I was aware that death was a realistic possibility because I remembered a woman who had lost her husband during his angiogram. His artery had ruptured and he didn't survive. I didn't want that to be me.

I also thought about the future. What if I did survive and ended up being this weak, pathetic, dependant person? Would I then just be a burden to my loved ones?

I *knew* that they would care for me, but at what cost to themselves? As difficult and poignant as it was to contemplate the possibility that I may perhaps die, the notion of being a burden to my family was even more distressing to me. What did my future, if there was one, hold?

In my quest for answers, I couldn't help but think about all those people out there who didn't even *try* to take care of themselves. Some ate as they pleased and smoked and drank to excess. Some lived a party lifestyle and did drugs. Where were they *right* now? They were home sleeping in their snug little beds. They weren't in CCU as I was, staring down the barrel of an angiogram. It made me feel so frustrated and angry! It didn't make sense to me. I wanted it to be *them* and not *me*. I had honestly tried to do what was right. *I didn't deserve this.* I guess this was my version of, "why me."

I'm a practical person, I always have been. So I thought about the financial aspect. What was this going to mean for my family financially? We did have health insurance, but I knew that medical costs could sometimes cause financial ruin for a family. I didn't want that either. I knew that I had no choice right now, but I figured by this point, I must have *at least* satisfied my deductible. I couldn't dwell on this. I'd have to think of something else right now. It's very upsetting that money has to be a concern at such a critical point in our lives.

All these darting thoughts and wild rantings were broken up periodically by several breaks to answer the call of nature. As I mentioned earlier, in the emergency room, the nurse gave me an injection of a diuretic. It was now working and required *repeated* calls to the nurse.

The nurse informed me that I would have to use the bedpan, since I wasn't allowed to get up. *Oh, joy of joys!* This is *not* an easy task if you are not used to it, and I hope that it's something I never "get used to." I don't know why I wasn't allowed to use a bedside potty. It felt like such a strain on me and my heart to try to use the bedpan, I could feel my chest tighten and my arms tremble. I honestly feel that this straining, in such a weakened condition, cannot possibly be good for your heart. I'm certain, if I were allowed the use of a bedside potty, this would have felt less stressful. I don't have a great deal of criticism, but perhaps whoever decides this, needs to rethink this one.

One relief I had was observing that my nurse was very germ conscious; this was comforting to me. I do have certain issues with germs, being a bit paranoid about them. I noticed that my nurse used gloves and she cleaned her hands with hand sanitizer, every time that she *entered* and *exited* the room. I did feel better about that, not that I was totally comfortable being in a hospital. A hospital, in my mind, is a place where you can get sicker than you were when you came in. You hear so much today about hospital-acquired infections being rampant. I was dealing with enough; I surely didn't need that.

Once again, I was alone with my thoughts in the silent darkness. I tried to relax, but was that even possible under the circumstances? I began to reflect on my life as a whole. My parents had brought me up to be a good person, with strong, core values. I wondered, "Had I lived up to those values? Had I made a good name with God and others?" I hoped that I had. I deeply felt that I had at least tried. I pondered, "What did people really think of me as a person? What if I did die, how would I be remembered? What would they say about me at my funeral?" This mélange of contemplations made me feel so anxious.

Sometimes it can be beneficial to reflect honestly on our lives. It can help us to see ourselves as we really are, so that we can adjust the things we don't like. I would however, recommend you doing this under different circumstances. You need to do this *before* you find yourself in a life or death situation. I concluded for the most part, I had few regrets about my life; there were at least, *no big regrets* I could recall. I guess at that point, I was trying to make peace with my inner self. All these recent events were still difficult for me to comprehend. I felt so weary! I was physically exhausted and mentally drained; I had not been able to sleep all that long, restless night.

CHAPTER 11

There were a few times I closed my eyes and as I did so, I tried to imagine that this must be a bad dream. I so very much *wanted* it to be a dream. I was trying to convince myself it just couldn't be real. Then my eyes would open, and I was faced with the stark reality of CCU, reminding me once again that I was not dreaming.

Two nurses, one male, one female, came in to prep me for the angiogram procedure. As demeaning as that was, it was a relief to have a break from my own anxious thoughts. They prepped my wrist and both sides of my groin by shaving the groin, and then scrubbing both areas with a sterilizing solution. With both sites prepped, the doctor could determine which site he would choose to use.

Looking back, I understand just how all of this may sound. You may be thinking that all my wild thoughts resemble the rantings of a crazy person. I now realize that too, as I relive these moments in my mind to put it on paper. It sounds like I perhaps needed to be in the mental health ward instead of CCU. It was just such a restless, distressing, traumatic night, coupled with the fact that I guess my imagination is just a *little* wilder than most.

You may also find that my attitude may seem a bit negative. I don't consider myself a negative person, and I don't want to be one. I think it was just the stress of a bad situation that brought out the worst in me. Under normal circumstances, I try to be a positive person, but I guess those who are around me on a regular basis would be the ones to ask about this. Even though I consider myself a positive person, I'm not one of those, "Pie in the sky" kind of people. You know the kind of person where everything is rainbows, butterflies, and cute little puppies. Those types really grate on your nerves and I think that most people would agree with that. I'm not the "Debbie Downer" type either; they can get on your last good nerve too. No one wants to be around people like that either. I would classify myself as a *realist*. I try to see things as they *really* are, and then work to make things better, if I possibly can. They say the pessimist sees the glass as half-empty and the optimist as half-full. If that is the case, the realist sees the spots left on the glass by the dishwasher (perhaps the realist and the perfectionist are closely related).

I feel it is important to be realistic about the things we face in life. Some people will say that *anyone* can do *anything* if they just put their minds to it. I don't agree. This is just a mantra that we as parents use to try to motivate our children, even though we know it's not entirely true. We've said it so often; we start to believe it ourselves. In reality no matter how hard we try, most of us have limitations. On the other hand, to go along with our limitations and weaknesses, we *all* have strengths. I think that it is better to concentrate on those strengths and work to develop and improve them. If we do, we'll get more benefit from our efforts and accomplish more good. That of course, is just one woman's opinion.

Since that long stressful night, I have come to one conclusion. I don't think I'm the only person who has ever been through this gamut of emotions. I am sure others; maybe many others, have felt all the same things I have described. At the time though, you do wonder to yourself, "Is this normal? Am I losing it?"

I honestly feel that all hospitals should have a therapist or counselor on staff, someone with specialized training who can be there for people in serious circumstances like this ... even if it's the middle of the night. I know I *really* needed someone to talk with about my fears, someone who understood what I was going through. I needed someone to tell me positive, soothing things like, "It's going to be okay," or to relate positive experiences of others in similar circumstances who have done well in the past. I *needed* someone who could say reassuring things at the right time. There is a proverb in the Bible found at Proverbs 25:11 (*NWT*) that says, "Like apples of gold in silver carvings is a word spoken at the right time." This I know is so true ... I desperately needed apples of gold that night.

I feel positive reinforcement at this time would lessen the stress that you experience initially. I don't see how those preliminary hours of emotional distress can be beneficial to your heart. Wouldn't this stress and anxiety put additional strain on your already weakened heart? Perhaps, couldn't that even trigger another cardiac event? Again, it is something to ponder.

It was *finally* morning. I hadn't slept, not a wink. The activity level was beginning to increase in CCU. What would this day bring for me? I was unsure, but I was hoping for the best. There was now a doctor at my bedside introducing himself to me, his name was Dr. Nair and he was the cardiologist on call. He was now *my cardiologist* and would be the doctor performing my angiogram. We discussed different matters related to the procedure.

He asked me, "Did you know that your cholesterol was high?" I told him that I did. He then asked me why I wasn't taking cholesterol medications.

"Because I was concerned about the side effects."

"I can assure you that the side effects of a heart attack are much worse than the side effects of cholesterol medication."

I couldn't argue with that logic because I knew and *agreed* that he was right. With an overview now of the big picture, I fully comprehend now just how *foolish* my reasoning was *and* must have sounded to my doctor.

He told me I would *now* have to regularly take medication for my heart, as well as cholesterol medication. He stressed the importance of my taking them correctly and consistently, and I promised to comply. I had learned my lesson; I try *not* to make the same mistakes twice. My only request was for him to consider being conservative in the medications that he selected to prescribe for me. I told him I was a conservative person and liked to start small. I asked him to please take that into consideration, he assured me he would do his best.

He confirmed that I was scheduled for 11:00 a.m. for the angiogram. After he left, I asked the nurse if he was a good doctor. I didn't know him; he was simply the cardiologist on call that morning. I realize now that question was somewhat silly on my part, as if she would have told me "no." She assured me that he was a very good doctor, with a good reputation. She told me all the cardiologists who were in the group were good doctors and that the cardiology firm is very selective. The doctors are carefully screened, only hiring the most qualified. That did make me feel a bit more reassured.

This cardiology group started here in my hometown. I even went to high school with its founder. These doctors are highly respected in the area. As a group, they have become world-renowned for treatment and research with people traveling great distances to see them. There is a *real need* for superior heart care in this area of South Louisiana. This is due to the fact that there is a prevalence of heart disease here, as I mentioned earlier. The nurse was *not* just saying nice things about my doctor to make me feel better, because since then I have heard nothing but good from others who have him as their doctor.

The next face I saw at my bedside was my family doctor, the one I had seen four days earlier. Someone from the hospital had notified him that I was in CCU. He looked very sheepish and told me, "I just didn't think it was your heart. I knew your age and your history, and I really didn't think it to be your heart."

He told me after the angiogram I would feel much better because I would be getting more oxygen if the heart attack was caused by a blockage. I don't harbor any ill feelings towards him. My case was not exactly typical and we all make mistakes. He did come to visit me every morning while I was in CCU (and no, he didn't charge me for those visits). He really did seem genuinely concerned about me.

Next, the nurse brought consent forms for me to sign. If you're not scared before you have read them, you will be after! I am probably one of the few people who actually took the time to thoroughly read this document. I knew its purpose—besides protecting the hospital and the doctor, a patient has to give informed consent. Informed consent implies that you know just what you are getting into, before you agree to the procedure. The nurse very casually explained the gist of what was on the pages. The risks start out simple, things like headache, nausea, or sore throat. They progressively get more serious. Next, you are reading about the possibility of stroke, heart attack, and *finally death.*

I was pretty sure those serious risks don't happen very often, and possibly wouldn't happen to me. It's just the fact that it's on the list, is proof that it can, and has happened in the past. What do you do? You want to say, "Hey, this is just too scary and risky. I don't want to sign this!" Of course, you know they won't proceed without your signature. They have to protect themselves too. I get that. *So* … with a deep, heavy sigh … I signed. All the while, I was praying that I wouldn't become that one in a million that those serious risks would affect.

The next face I see as she walks through the door is my beautiful mother. She is dressed in her navy pantsuit, looking like a billion bucks. She has her makeup on and every hair in place. Her mother stressed the importance of being neat and presentable when going places. My grandmother was always very particular about her appearance and passed on that message to the rest of the family. She went to the beauty shop every week to have her hair done and did this until she was hospitalized at ninety-eight years old. With her, it didn't have to be fancy or expensive, just clean, neat, and well arranged. She was so special to us all because she taught us so many valuable life lessons.

Here was my dear mother; worry evident on her face. She had the same wounded look that my daughter had earlier that morning. I hated to see her like this over me.

I smiled at her as she walked in and said, "Can you believe this?" Her look of anguish indicated that she did not.

She told me she was home getting ready, so that she could take me to my doctor's appointment as promised. That was when my sister arrived and broke the news to her saying, "I've got good news and bad news. The good news is you don't have to drive Kim to her doctor's appointment. The bad news is she is already in the hospital. She's had a heart attack, but she's okay."

Mother related that she had been shocked to hear the news, which was to be the repetitive response from everyone when they learned what had happened to me. I wasn't the typical person who looked like "a heart attack waiting to happen." My mother stayed at my bedside and I was glad the nurse allowed her to do so. It was just what I needed at that time. A girl needs her mother there to make her feel better, no matter how old she is.

My daughter had arrived from New Orleans by this time. I was relieved that she had arrived safely and was pleased that I could spend some time with her for a little while before my procedure as well. I had been worried about her rushing to see me. I was concerned that her mind would not be on her driving, but on me. My younger daughter had been in and out several times to check on me too. I could tell that she *really* did not want to be at work that day. There were thoughts of a serious nature that I contemplated bringing up. The, "What if I don't make it" talk ... but I decided not to go there. I didn't want to create any additional stress other than what they already were dealing with. I told them all that I loved them, but they already knew that because I tell them all the time anyway. Life is just too short and too fragile not to tell those we care about, just how much we love them! *That* was by far the most important thing they needed to know at this time.

I have a close friend who lives in Georgia that I tried to call, but I got her answering machine. I had really hoped to talk to her, but I didn't want to leave a negative message on her machine and alarm her. I just told her that I had something to tell her. I told her to call my daughter's phone because, "I would be out of pocket for a while." Boy, was that the understatement of the year.

CHAPTER 12

Next, one of the nurses from the cath lab came to see me. He wanted to give me a brief idea of what was going to take place during the angiogram. He was extremely personable and *VERY* handsome. In fact, I would later learn that many of the hospital staff were simply *"ga ga"* over him. Just let me say this... he makes George Clooney look like sloppy seconds. Of course, I understand that his appeal is, however, very limited—that is, limited to the ladies in the 18-80 age group. Just looking at him made you feel so much better, a *very* handy attribute for a nurse to have, I might add. For anonymity's sake, I will just nickname him George. He left and then shortly returned and told me he was coming to take me to the catheterization (cath) lab. This was earlier than I had expected to go. My husband was not back yet (we told him that the procedure was scheduled for 11:00 a.m.). I guess an opening in the schedule came up earlier than anticipated. I felt *panicked*! George proceeded to get me ready to go. He was in a cheerful mood for it being so early in the morning. As we left CCU, he was pushing the gurney very fast and making crazy turns.

"I feel like I'm on Mr. Toad's Wild Ride!" I told him.

"This is the most dangerous part of the procedure," he replied. "If you survive the gurney ride to the cath lab, you'll be fine. I'm better at doing my job in the cath lab, than I am at driving gurneys," he assured.

Just outside of CCU, my mother was waiting alone. I asked George if we could stop for a minute in order to call my husband and he was nice enough to do this for me. I told my husband they were taking me early. He said he was on his way back and he loved me. I knew he was upset that he didn't get to see me before going to the cath lab, but I told him I was going to be okay, to be careful, and that I loved him.

After kissing my mother and telling her I loved her, I was on my way to the cath lab. Of the millions of thoughts that I could have been thinking right then, why was I thinking negative thoughts? I couldn't stop thinking about the man mentioned earlier, the one whose artery ruptured during his angiogram, and who didn't survive. I tried to put that thought far out of my mind, a task easier said than done. I tried to change the subject.

My next "pressing" thought, was my full bladder. I told George I was sorry that I had not used the bedpan before leaving for the cath lab. My diuretics evidently were still working. He told me once we got to the back; there was a restroom that I could use. I thought, "A real restroom, not a bedpan? Oh, be still my pathetic, beating heart!" George pushed the gurney into the narrow hallway outside of the cath lab suite. The door across the hallway was to an employee's restroom.

I was allowed to go in by myself, which surprised me. For the second time that day, I grabbed the back of my lovely open-backed gown. I went in, but didn't lock the door in case I got weak or worse—passed out. I wanted to be sure that help could quickly arrive if I needed it. There I was, in an employee rest room that also doubled as a storage closet for supplies. I was nervous and apprehensive as to what my future held. So what did I do? I took the time to spread paper on the toilet seat before sitting down, just as I always do on public toilets. Mama had taught me well ... and I guess old habits *are* hard to break.

Thinking back, it was somewhat funny. If I was going to live, I certainly didn't want to "catch something" from a hospital toilet seat. Who knows what kinds of germs are on there? It was wonderful to sit on a real toilet instead of a bedpan. It's the sort of thing that makes you realize that you should *never* take the little things for granted. I washed my hands, went out, and got back on the gurney.

Next, George pushed the gurney into the room where the angiogram was going to take place. It was a large, cool, dimly lit room with the exception of a few strategically placed spot-type lights. There were five to six people in the room (all men). They were nurses and technicians; however, I am not sure who was who. At the south end of the room, there was a wall of glass. Behind it was the control room. Inside were men sitting at computers facing me. Their job was to process and record the pictures and information obtained during the angiogram. I had to transfer from the gurney to the X-ray table—a very hard, narrow table. I tried to *scoot* from the gurney to the table. This sounds very simple, but it was a tricky feat. Please allow me to explain. There I was a *woman* wearing a short, open-backed gown and no underwear. As I have just explained, the men in the control room were facing me behind the wall of glass. I tried to *scoot* in the most lady-like manner that I could, all the while holding my gown down and trying not to expose myself. It was, in short, an athletic feat. I can only hope that I executed it well. If there was such a sport as "Gurney Scooting"—I would like to think that I could have scored a 10.0.

All the guys back there had this great sense of humor and were so nice. The overall mood was very tranquil as they went about their individual jobs in a calm and relaxed manner. This, I must say helped to put me more at ease. Most of them have been working together for many years, so there was a certain cohesiveness to the way they work with one another. I knew this was routine for them, but it certainly wasn't for me. I told them I was scared. They reassured me that I was going to be fine, that I was in good hands. One of the nurses stood on my right side. He went through a standard checklist they ask all patients before sedation is administered. Questions like: Do you wear dentures? Do you wear contacts? Do you have sleep apnea? "No, no, no."

My left arm was stretched out and strapped down. They would attempt to go in through the left radial artery. I preferred that to an incision in the groin. Above me, there was a large device, The Image Intensifier: an X-ray camera that would be taking pictures of my heart. While this was above me, the X-ray beam was to be delivered from underneath the table through an X-ray tube. Images were going to be live on the monitor above me, and were to be recorded on a computer disc drive as well. The X-ray tube and Image Intensifier were to be rotated around me in different directions. By doing this, the cardiologist could inspect blockages from several different projections, enabling him to make a more accurate assessment of the issues affecting my heart. In turn, that would help him in determining the most effective method of treatment. The room was kept dimly lit to make the monitor screen more visible.

I was informed that I was going to be given sedation soon. Sedation is different from general anesthesia. With general anesthesia, the patient is in a deep coma-like sleep where they experience loss of motor reflexes and total relaxation. The type of sedation that I was to be given is known as conscious sedation. These types of intravenous medications are used to create a state of overall relaxation for the patient. A most important benefit of conscious sedation is that the patient, although seemingly asleep, is able to follow instructions. Patients, for instance, may be asked to take a deep breath or to cough. Coughing can improve the quality of the pictures or bring the heart back to a normal rhythm if there is an arrhythmia. There are different levels of sedation and some patients are more conscious than others are. I feel free to assume that the level is determined by how nervous they sense the patient to be. Some patients remember what took place during their procedure, and some do not. They apparently chose to knock me out completely. I told them, "Take good care of me." I realized I was about to be sedated and with my last cognizant thought, I remember supplicating God in prayer... pleading that if I did not survive, to *please* help my family to cope with the loss. *They* were my main concern right now.

*Fade to **black**,...*

and... LIGHTS ᴏᴜᴛ!

CHAPTER 13

Fast-forward two and a half hours. My first conscious thought was, "*Oh, my back hurts so much.*" I had been on that narrow, hard table for such a long time. I initially realized that they were still working on me, because I could hear them talking and then noticed the screen above me. I could see the wire moving in my heart, which was absolutely amazing! I have always been enamored with programs on television that featured actual surgery since I found them to be so interesting. This show was live and I had a front row seat. What was even better was ... *my heart* was the star of *this* show! It dawned on me, "Hey, I'm alive! I made it." I was elated!

I felt so thirsty though. I felt as if I had been in a desert for days. I had never been that parched before. I asked if someone could wipe my mouth with a wet cloth and someone came to my aid right away. The cool cloth on my lips felt so soothing. I was still thirsty, but it helped somewhat. I was emerging from my drug-induced stupor and becoming more alert. That is another benefit of conscious sedation; patients are able to recover from it rapidly. I realized that my left wrist felt sore. Before I was sedated, they had told me they planned to enter through the left wrist for the procedure; that was plan A. They had prepped my groin as well; that was plan B. From where they were standing, I could tell that they were working from the artery in my groin. One of the nurses told me that the doctor wasn't able to get to where he needed to be through the radial artery in my arm. Therefore, it was necessary to go through the right femoral artery in my groin. They were almost finished with the procedure and I was informed that I had blockages that were fixed with stents. I thought, "So I did have a blockage after all." Remembering back to the emergency room, I had doubts as to whether this would be the case. At the time, I felt like if I had blockages, I would know. I guess that idea was blown out of the water.

I next found out that, I had in fact, had *four* blockages that needed stents and they were in the process of finishing the third one. One of the nurses told me that the contrast dye used in the angiogram is hard on the kidneys. In order to prevent kidney damage they wanted to limit my time with the contrast dye in my system. They were planning to open and stent the final blockage on Thursday (it was still Tues*day*, a very long day— probably the longest day of my life). That would give me time to void the dye, so that my kidneys could recover. My doctor also wanted me to rest so that my heart failure could improve.

I was glad all had gone well, but I now had another angiogram hanging over my head. The *thought* of having another angiogram in two days was most unsettling to me. Nevertheless, what choice did I have? Finishing touches on the procedure were completed and I was back on the gurney, being wheeled towards CCU by George. As he pushed me through the large double doors, we could hear the roar of many excited voices.

"What is all of that?" He said.

I recognized the noisy din coming from the CCU waiting area and proudly claimed them as my own.

"That's my family." I confessed, "We refer to ourselves as the 'Loud Family' like on Saturday Night Live."

As he pushed me past the waiting area door, there was a clamor of excitement. These were my family and friends—my people. I had my own entourage. A sizable group had come to be together to wait and wish me well.

Doctor Oz asks his patients before surgery, "Who loves you and who do you love?" He says if your heart doesn't have a reason to keep beating, it won't. I knew as I looked into their faces that I had so many wonderful reasons for my heart to keep beating. It was evident that so many people loved and cared about me. I was delighted beyond words to see everyone and excitedly told them all, to come and follow me; I was going back to my room. It seemed as if I *thought* I was hosting a giant "I'm Alive" party.

Someone spoke up and said, "She's back to normal, she's barking orders again."

Everyone laughed and someone commented on how alert I was to which George responded, "I know, and we gave her enough drugs to knock out a small water buffalo." He sounded amazed.

I was happy! I was back among the living again. George brought me back to CCU and settled me in. I guess the party would have to wait because I was only allowed *one* visitor. Mother came back to sit at my bedside. George said that I would have to lie *flat* for the next six hours. I was not supposed to raise my head so as not to put pressure on the opening in my groin. It's not a very big incision; however, it's not sutured closed. For the first twenty minutes, manual, physical pressure would be exerted at the incision site. The person in charge of that job? *That's right*, it was George!

Once I was settled again in CCU, George removed the sheath from my incision site that had held the catheter. It's necessary to press down and hold this area with firm pressure for the entire time. He frequently had to change hands in order to keep a steady, firm pressure on the site, which must have been very difficult. I can only imagine how tired his hands must have gotten. I asked why they don't suture the incision closed. He told me the artery is very elastic and seals itself when the sheath is removed. The physical pressure at the site, allows time for a clot to form. This is why no stitches are necessary. I just needed to lie still so that the clot is not disturbed. This is especially important since I was given multiple blood thinners in preparation for the angiogram. I later learned that my daughter told some of her co-workers about this. When they learned that it was George holding my groin, she said there were several who volunteered to swap places with me for my *next* angiogram. I recall thinking that I really *wished* they could.

I remember telling my mother, "I'm so grateful to be alive and grateful they were able to resolve my issues without open-heart surgery." I really didn't want that! Just the thought of having my chest opened and my ribs spread made me shudder. I knew that it must be extremely painful and I had experienced *enough* pain in the last two weeks to last me a lifetime.

I noticed that my head was hurting and mentioned it to George. He told me that the nitroglycerin patch applied to my chest in the cath lab caused the headache. Nitroglycerin works by relaxing and widening blood vessels so that blood can flow more easily to the heart. He reassured me that the headache was normal.

I asked my mother if she had talked with the cardiologist after my procedure. I wanted an update on what had actually transpired during the angiogram, before I woke up. She then showed me the diagram that they make for the patients. (See page 238) It's a drawing of the heart that shows the various coronary arteries. It shows the location of the blockages and stent placement, as well as the percentages of the blockages.

There was a 99% blockage in the Left Anterior Descending artery (referred to as the LAD). Doctors commonly refer to a heart attack that results from a proximal blockage in the LAD, as "the widow-maker." I guess in women, it would be called "the widow*er*-maker." Blockage to this artery is dramatic because the LAD supplies blood to the major vessels of the heart, feeding the bulk of the heart muscle. The LAD supplies blood to the front of the left ventricle (LV) and the partition wall that separates the LV from the right ventricle (RV). The LV is the most important pumping chamber of the heart because it supplies oxygenated blood to the body.

I also had a 99% and a 70% blockage in the Circumflex artery (CIRC). The CIRC wraps around the heart and supplies blood to the back wall of the LV. This was where the blockages were opened and three stents placed today. On Thursday, the last blockage was going to be addressed. It was a 90% blockage in the Right Coronary artery (RCA). The RCA supplies blood to the bottom wall of the LV, as well as, supplying branches of the RV.

Looking at the diagram, I also saw that there were two other blockages to a lesser degree in the LAD and the RCA. There were two blockages as well, in the distal subsections of the LAD and the CIRC. These are blockages that are located at the bottom of the heart where the artery narrows and cannot be opened with stents. In fact, they don't make stents small enough to open these. I wondered how my heart could have developed these extents of blockages in only 55 years. I was *shocked* that all three of the main arteries of my heart were involved, and that the blockages were so significant. My heart was literally *starving* for blood.

I would learn that the stents I had received were drug-eluding stents. A drug-eluding stent has a time-release medication embedded in it that slowly releases into the area around the stent. This medication works to help prevent blockages from building up inside the stent. This works in conjunction with an anti-platelet medication that I would be taking orally.

These stents differed from the stents put in place for my father eighteen years earlier. The earlier versions were a tremendous break-through, at that time. They saved many lives. However, they were not drug-eluding and didn't work as well as the ones that are available today. The older versions tended to block up more easily. I was *relieved* to have this procedure successfully behind me, but still in disbelief at the extent of the blockages.

At least I had an answer to my question of *why*. Now I knew exactly what had caused my heart attack, but two 99% blockages, a 90%, and a 70% blockage? It's little wonder that I had been in so much pain. The thing that was so mind boggling to me was, for two weeks prior to the heart attack, I would have pain and then it would get better for a little while, and then I would be in severe pain again. I always thought that when you had a heart attack threatening, the pain and symptoms would come on suddenly and continue to get progressively worse in a short span of time *and* there would be chest pain. At that point, you would realize that something was terribly wrong, and you would know that you needed to go to the hospital *or* died on the spot. I certainly was glad it wasn't the latter.

I mistakenly thought that because your symptoms were not constant and would seem to go away, that meant that you weren't experiencing something serious like a heart attack and didn't have to be *as* concerned. I guess like most people, I had in mind the "Hollywood Heart Attack." We've seen it portrayed so many times on television we think *that* is what a heart attack is really like. My symptoms were not nearly so dramatic or impressive. Still I wondered how I could have *not* discerned what was taking place. I thought I was a person who was in tune with my body. Perhaps I didn't realize because I didn't have what *I* thought to be, the "textbook" heart attack. It's mainly because of the fact that a heart attack can present itself in an *obscure* way that I have endeavored to write with so many details. I hope that if anyone starts to experience something similar, I trust you will make the connection that I simply did not.

My younger daughter popped in again for a short visit to check on me. She was so relieved that all had gone well and looked so much better than the worried girl that I saw earlier that morning. She relayed to me that the cardiologist had said it was a good thing I had not been a smoker. If I had smoked, I may not have made it. *Many people who have heart attacks that result from a significant blockage in their LAD do not get a second chance.* I had been very fortunate indeed!

My twenty minutes of compression on my incision were over, but I still had to lie flat so as not to open the wound. I bid George farewell for today. My mother next noticed that she could see a dramatic improvement in my coloring. She said earlier, I had a grey cast to my skin and I now looked a lot pinker. It's amazing what a sufficient amount of oxygen will do for your countenance.

The nurse finally brought me ice chips. I had been craving ice or water since I was in the cath lab. I wasn't allowed to have it too soon, to lessen the chance of nausea and vomiting. They wisely wanted to avoid that. I first got ice chips and then I graduated to cold water. I savored it like it was the best water I had ever tasted. It felt as if I could not get enough to quench my thirst and *thankfully*, it agreed with me and stayed down. The nurse now *encouraged* me to drink in order to help flush out the contrast dye from my body.

Next, I had a new and interesting challenge. You may find it odd that I am including things of a seemingly trivial nature. Even so, I just wanted to portray the full *hospital experience* by including the menial details as well. These are the things that nobody even gives a thought to … until faced with them. I needed to use the bedpan and buzzed for the nurse. She told me she'd help me, but that I couldn't sit up or strain because of the incision in my groin, I'd have to remain *completely* flat. This was to prevent the incision from starting to bleed. I was puzzled and asked,

"How do I use the bedpan *without* sitting up?"

"*Very carefully*," she replied.

And, the procedure went like this:
She rolled me over on the opposite side from the incision, all the while not lifting my head and keeping my body completely straight. Next, a thin bedpan was slid under me. I was then, rolled back over, flat on my back—ready ... get set ... go ...

I can attest that this is *not* an easy thing to do because you don't have the advantage of gravity. Even though you *really* have to go, you have to *concentrate* very hard. I asked the nurse for a little time and privacy. The task takes place in increments, but after some time, the mission is finally accomplished.

The *next trick* is being rolled back over in order to remove the bedpan, except this time, the bedpan is stuck to your bottom and filled with liquid. The nurse next endeavors to *carefully* separate the two, without spilling anything, another feat in itself. Only another human who has been through this would understand just how uncomfortable, humiliating, and difficult this is. The other problem is that you have to repeat this ordeal quite a few times in the six hours that you are in this prone position. *And* you are given another diuretic to encourage the voiding of the contrast dye from the angiogram.

The rest of the afternoon was fairly uneventful. It was about time for some normalcy in my life. I really needed that now. I was able to rest and relax a bit. I don't remember going to sleep though, the only "sleep" that I got that day was during the angiogram.

CHAPTER 14

As I lie there, I mulled over the morning's events. I hoped that I wasn't in any impending danger, while awaiting the second angiogram. I knew they had fixed the most crucial areas first. At any rate, if something did go wrong, I was in the best possible place. At least I was being constantly monitored.

I thought about my blockages. I felt responsible. I reproached myself first for not heeding the doctor's advice about taking the cholesterol medication. If *only* I had *listened*; I wouldn't be in this situation. I might not have developed blockages, but I felt I knew better. I had let other people's opinions sway my judgment. If only I could go back and do it all over again, but we all know, there are no "do-overs" in life. I remember thinking, "I only wish I could go back in time, to before the heart attack, *then* I would be okay." However, that line of reasoning was only an illusion. I wasn't really okay before the heart attack; I just thought that I was, when in fact, I had four significant blockages. I *couldn't* turn the clock back; I would have to move forward.

The other thing I had deep regrets about was not recognizing that my symptoms were heart related. I blamed myself and was angry for not realizing it. I thought I knew and understood my own body, but I had allowed it to deceive me. I did tell myself that my family doctor had missed it too, and that helped a little bit. I was now *finally* realizing that I had misinterpreted my many symptoms. I had conveniently blamed old injuries for the cause of my pain and that was the reason I denied and dismissed what I was feeling. However, I would in the future, forgive myself for both of these mistakes. In reality, not recognizing the symptoms in advance of the heart attack was actually a blessing in disguise, but I'll expound on this a little later in my story.

A sonographer came to CCU to perform an echocardiogram. An echocardiogram is simply an ultrasound study that produces images of the heart. This is such a useful tool because it can *non-invasively* determine heart structure and the location of damaged portions of the heart muscle. It measures the strength of the heart, in addition to blood flow and uses Doppler to measure the velocity of blood flow in certain areas of the heart. I asked the technician if he could reveal any of his findings, but he said he couldn't, the doctor would have to review the results and would then let me know.

It was now suppertime. As my meal was delivered, I discovered that I was on a cardiac/diabetic diet. Which translated, means low salt, low fat/cholesterol, and low carbs. This also translates into *no taste.* Even though it had been many hours since I had eaten, I didn't feel very hungry so I ate just a small portion. It was then and there that I made a promise to myself. As I stared at my supper, I knew that my diet had probably played some part, maybe a *big* part, in my blockages. I knew that I had made some improvements in the last two years, but what about the other fifty-three years?

When you're younger, you don't realize that your bad habits are going to catch up with you, at least not so quickly. You have this idea that you are totally invincible and you think you have a long time before you need to make changes. As every middle-aged person will tell you, it comes much faster than you think it will. You get involved with your life and the fast pace of living, and all of a sudden you realize that you need to take better care of yourself. The problem being, what kind of damage did you do in the time in between? Most people probably eat well up until their teenage years, and then good nutrition goes out the window. I remember as a teen, my mother *really tried* to teach me about nutrition. She cooked good, healthy meals for us, but what did I do? I ate lemon cookies for breakfast. Had all those lemon cookies come back to haunt me? Was *this* the ghosts of cookies past?

It was in those moments, as I stared at my dinner tray, that I promised myself I was going to make real and lasting changes. Even more changes than I had made before, and I was going to stick to it. I was going to eat as if my life depended on it because I knew *now* it did. The fact that, for the most part, I had lost my appetite early on, made this promise easier to keep. I made up my mind that this *wasn't* going to be *just* a diet, but now my *new way of life*. Nowadays, when people ask how I lost my weight, I tell them I'm on the Heart Attack Diet. When they ask, "What does that consist of?" I tell them, to take away the salt, the fat and the sugar from their diet and the food will taste so *bland*, that they'll only want to eat very small portions. I promise that you will lose weight with this regimen!

That same night, I was allowed to have visitors in CCU. My family and friends were all so pleased to hear that I was doing better. I finally remembered I had planned to go to a painting class that night, with a friend. She came to see me in CCU and I told her that I didn't really think I would be able to attend the class tonight. She said she would let me off until another time.

I told my family that it had occurred to me that I *now* had no chance of realizing one of my goals. I was an avid *Survivor* fan and I had been since the beginning. I was very intrigued with the whole concept of the show and wished that I could be a player. My sister felt the same way and we would have made a tremendous team. I didn't necessarily think that I could win; I just would have liked the opportunity to play the game. After all, they always had at least one *obligatory* older woman. I felt that I could've held my own, at least for a while. A strong Cajun woman has many skills that could benefit a player, as we are extremely resilient, resourceful people. I was now painfully aware that dream would never come to pass because of my heart issues. I knew that it was a silly pipe dream, but now it was one less pipe dream for me. I probably wouldn't have been able to leave my family for thirty-nine days, even if I had been accepted to play. Thus, all in all, I guess it didn't really matter. I did have something to look forward to though; after all, *Survivor* was coming back on television in less than a month.

Many months later, as I thought back to that night, an "*ah ha*" thought hit me and I came to a new realization about this matter. While I would never play the game seen on television, I *had* in actuality, played the game in *real life*. I had in effect, won immunity that day in the cath lab, and I was given the chance to stay in the game a little longer. *I* was a *real life* survivor! There was *still* fire in my torch ... the cardiologist had spoken! There was no million-dollar prize at the end, but I had something better.

After visiting hours ended, my friends and family went home for the night. I was astonished to learn that I was to be the *guest of honor* at a basic hospital activity. This would be the *infamous* hospital bath. I must say I've engaged in activities that I've enjoyed more. A long time ago, I had heard it said, "When you check into the hospital, you need to check your modesty at the door. You can then pick it up on your way out." This of course, is more easily said, than done. The kind nurse from the night before was back and she was in charge of the bathing with the help of an aide. She did her best to be quick and professional. I was embarrassed, but I got through it. I normally enjoy a good bath, but I do hope that I *never* need to do that again.

I was clean and my sheets were fresh, maybe I could finally get some rest. At this time, I had been in the hospital about twenty hours, not even a full day. *So much* had happened in such a short time. I was still thinking about the events that had taken place that day, but I was much calmer now and I felt *truly* grateful to be alive. I tried to watch television for a little while, but I couldn't concentrate because it was *still* difficult to turn my mind off.

The nurse came in and offered me a sleeping pill, saying that the doctor had left orders for one if I needed it. As I said earlier, I don't like to take pills, but I accepted. I knew that I needed the rest since I hadn't slept at all the night before. I was able go to sleep, but I was still somewhat restless, waking up many times during the night.

CHAPTER 15

Wednesday, August 17, 2011

I awoke the next morning, happy and thankful to be a part of this new day. It was going to be my lazy day, my day off. This was to be my lazy day on the Lazy Lagoon that was long overdue, minus the sun, the water, and the inner tube of course. My doctor had told me it was a chance for me to rest up and allow my kidneys to recover before my next angiogram, which was to be done the following day.

Since I seemed to be doing well, my nurse was again lenient with my visitors and I had company in and out all day long. As I had mentioned earlier, CCU tries to limit visitors to two at a time, but at times, they would break the rule for me. That made me happy because I *needed* my loved ones near me at this uncertain time in my life. My friends and family were all so supportive and caring. I was allowed to keep my cell phone, and I received many calls from well-wishers from Georgia to Montana. It felt good to know that so many were concerned about my welfare; I felt so loved.

That night, my older daughter and my dear friend were my last two visitors before visiting hours ended. They were getting ready to go home. I was giving my daughter some last minute instructions about the house and double-checking that the cat had been getting her medicine. I was still trying to run my house from a bed in CCU. She reassured me not to worry because she had *everything* under control. Just before it was time for them to leave, my new nurse came in. He told me that after my visitors left, he would come in to give me my bath and change my bed. *WHAT?* I just couldn't imagine having a male nurse bath me. I had met my quota for humiliation the night before. The only way this would have been okay with me was if my procedure the day before, had been a lobotomy instead of an angiogram.

I looked squarely at him and shook my head from side to side saying, "Please don't take this the wrong way, but I'm still a modest person. If you'll bring all the stuff, my friend and my daughter will help me with my bath and even change my sheets. They'll do *all* your work for you."

"Oh, I'm sorry Ms. Kim; I'm not used to my patients being conscious here in CCU. You are much more alert than the majority of my patients. I'd be glad to get everything for you so that your family can help you; I didn't mean to embarrass you," he said.

He brought everything in and my daughter and friend helped me with my "sink bath." One *awkward* bath had been enough for this hospital stay! I was reassured of just how much my friend loved me since she was willing to help me with a bath. My friend proved she was a true-blue friend that night.

Everyone went home and I tried to settle down for the night. I noticed a woman, who worked there at the hospital, walk past the glass front of my room several times. She looked familiar; I thought perhaps she was the daughter of a woman I knew. The next time she walked past my room, I motioned for her to come in and found out that she was indeed the person I thought she was.

We started to talk, she inquired about my health and I told her that I was there because of a heart attack. She asked, "Is this your first heart attack?" I was so taken aback by that question. *My first heart attack?* Was I to expect more? I *didn't* like the way that sounded. She told me that she had a heart attack several years back in her early forties. I inquired about *all* the details. She said she was fine, but she needed to quit smoking. I couldn't believe it! She had *survived* a heart attack and was still smoking?

I told her, "Yes, you do need to quit. Do you want to be in the place that I'm in right now?"

I *now* had a new mission, getting everyone else to take better care of themselves. I must say, it is encouraging to speak with someone who has survived the very thing that you are going through. I hung on her every word. It gave me *"hope"* that if she survived, I could too. The woman I spoke with that night did have another heart attack ten months later. I'm happy to say that she did survive *again*.

I was able to rest somewhat during the night, but as most people will tell you, hospitals are *not* easy places to rest. They can be *very* noisy. I was concerned about the angiogram the next day. It weighed heavily on my mind, but I was *not* as nervous as I was while waiting for the first one.

CHAPTER 16

Thursday, August 18, 2011

Morning had arrived—of course the day starts very early in a hospital. There was to be no breakfast for me this morning because of the angiogram. The angiogram was scheduled for 9:00 a.m. I was anxious to have it over and behind me, but I was still scared. The nurse brought in another consent form for me to sign since this was a separate procedure. For a second time, I was reminded of the dangers of just what can go wrong, but once more, I sighed, signed and hoped for the best.

In all the excitement of the past few days, I had forgotten something—my daughter's incident at the water park. I had made an appointment for her with a cardiologist for today. *She* was supposed to see a cardiologist today, not *me*. Life does take some interesting twists sometimes, does it not? I knew I would have to reschedule that appointment for her.

My family was back again that morning to support me. The angiogram was on schedule. George came to get me once again. As he rolled me back to the cath lab, he said he had a surprise for me and he introduced me to the newest member of their team. *Finally*, I wasn't alone; there was another female in the cath lab.

I told her, "I bet they give you a rough time back here, they seem like they could be a bunch of jokesters." She just smiled.

Again, here I was being prepped for the main event and I was covered with a sterile drape. This time the incision was going to be in my left femoral artery. I guess they sensed that I was not as nervous this time. For my "conscious sedation," this time, I was *actually* conscious. Since they had performed the first angiogram only two days earlier, they already had their game plan. It was now game time.

A numbing medication was inserted just below the skin, but I felt no physical discomfort. After making a small incision in my left femoral artery where it comes close to the surface of the skin, they inserted a small needle into the femoral artery. Next, a thin wire was inserted through this needle. Once the wire is in place, a small plastic catheter known as an "introducer," was then advanced over the wire. The introducer has a one-way valve that allows the introduction of additional catheters, while preventing backflow bleeding. The catheter, a thin, hollow, flexible tube was then slowly and gently guided toward my heart, into the aorta and into the openings of the coronary arteries. This is done with the assistance of fluoroscopic guidance. Fluoroscopy is a technique that uses X-ray to visualize moving structures in real time, similar to an X-ray movie. A small amount of dye was injected through the catheter and as it's injected and moves through your bloodstream, you feel a *warm* sensation. This dye is what allows the doctor to assess the presence and severity of blockages and also allows your arteries to be photographed by X-ray.

It had been previously determined that there was a 90% blockage in my Right Coronary artery (RCA). The objective was to open the blockage with what is commonly known as balloon angioplasty. At the tip of the catheter is a tiny balloon. Once it's in the correct location, the balloon is inflated. When this takes place, the balloon compresses the plaque up against the wall of the artery. This makes the opening inside the artery larger, to increase blood flow. Now that this area is opened, the stent is then expanded inside the once blocked area and left in place to keep the artery from narrowing or closing again. This procedure is called percutaneous transluminal coronary angioplasty (PTCA). This procedure, in my opinion, is *wonderful* because it can restore arterial blood flow to the heart *without* the need for open-heart surgery.

I was watching the monitor above me and seeing this entire procedure taking place—LIVE. It seems truly *amazing* to know how far technology has progressed in the field of cardiac medicine. These tiny, metal, wire-mesh tubes are now a *permanent* part of me. I guess you could say they're my new best friends, all four of them. I now wear my "bling" on the inside. Within a few days, the stent will start the process of being covered with tissue. I'll need to take anti-platelet medication for a length of time to lessen the chance of blood clots forming inside the stents. Anti-platelet medication makes the platelets "less sticky." This helps them to not clump together to form clots.

My procedure was complete and has been a success. My visit to the cath lab was of a much shorter duration today, only about forty minutes. I was so pleased that it was all behind me *finally* and that there had been such success. I felt that I could now *officially* start the recovery process.

George brought me back to CCU. We had to go through the same procedure as two days earlier, manual pressure on the incision site for twenty minutes again. My husband sat at my bedside this time. As we visited with George, we learned that his in-laws lived right around the corner from our home. It's a small world after all. We talked about everything from his dog waking him up before his clock went off, to how I make my iced tea. He's such a nice guy, truly an *asset* to the cath lab team. Even my husband liked him. I again, had to lie flat for the next six hours, just as before and yes, more bedpan breaks flat on my back. I did try to hold it as long as possible.

Later that evening, I think around 7:00 p.m., the nurse let me know that I was going to be transferred to a regular room. I wasn't expecting to be moved at that time, I thought it would be the next morning. I was just starting to feel more comfortable now that my procedures were behind me. I had been in this close, secure environment for three days and I felt *safe* in this womb-like place. I had just had a serious procedure hours earlier. I didn't really want to be moved, but evidently, my doctor thought I was well enough to go. In actuality, I really was ready *physically*, but *not* emotionally.

CHAPTER 17

My husband, my mother, and my two daughters were with me. I was transferred to a gurney for transport. I have to say, things can take on a different perspective when you're transported in a prone position. I'll try to explain. As I was being wheeled to my new room, my wild imagination was evidently wilder than ever.

Mostly, what you can see from this position is row after row of fluorescent lights. You also hear the consistent clicking of the gurney wheels. It's almost the same sound that the wheels make on a bad shopping cart. It's eerily reminiscent of a scene from a B-movie. You know the movie; it's the one where the deranged person is wheeling the helpless, semi-drugged woman down the hall to do no telling what. *Yeah, that movie!* All that she is able to see is out of focus, and a blur of row, after row, of dimly lit fluorescent lights speeding by.

Yes, I know it sounds crazy, but I had been through so much the past few days. This had been the most stressful event that I had yet faced. My life had been turned upside down, and here I was leaving the *one* place that I felt safe. When a person has any procedure that involves the heart, it can make them more emotional than usual. I would certainly testify to this fact. I would not doubt that the plethora of drugs over the past few days might have played *some* part as well.

Next, to add insult to injury, I was pushed down to the last room at the end of the hall. I felt like I was so isolated down there because I was so far from the nurse's station. I thought, "What if I need help?" It wasn't *anything* like it was in CCU. I should've been thrilled, the last room on the hall is the least noisy, but I didn't think of that. My family was discussing who was going to stay with me for the night. That was so caring and generous of them, but I could see in their faces how tired they all were. They had been through the mill for the last few days too. I think that it is sometimes harder on the family than on the patient, because your loved ones worry and feel so helpless in this sort of situation. I tried to pretend that I was going to be fine and *insisted* that they all go home to get a good night's rest. They wanted to stay, but I *finally* convinced them and they went home for the night. They had all been so wonderful. I really hoped that they could rest since the worst was now finally over.

This sounds so silly, but my next trepidation was with my new nurse. Poor guy, he turned out to be just great. If you can though, bear in mind that I was *not* in a good frame of mind at this time. At first, I didn't think that he looked like he was a nurse. Please don't misunderstand; there wasn't anything wrong with him. He just looked different from the concept of the caring nurturer that I had fixed in my head. He was a stocky, muscular type with a ruddy complexion and had a gruff, gravel voice. He looked more as if he would be a landscaper or a buff fireman than a nurse. He got me settled and tried to make me comfortable. He told me if I needed anything, just to buzz him.

I thought that I would watch a little television and I flipped through the channels. While I was doing this, I could hear loud voices. I turned the television down and tried to understand what was being said, but I could not. It got quiet again. I again tried to find some nice, wholesome show on television that would calm and entertain me, but could find nothing that fit that description. I felt on edge and uneasy. I decided to turn the television off and just try to relax. When I did so, I could hear the loud voice again. I still couldn't understand what was being said, but just the fact that it was continuing, made me very uncomfortable. It sounded like it was coming from the room next door, and someone sounded angry.

When I was in CCU, my husband had brought me a book from home, in case I wanted to read. I thought, "I'll just start that book." A friend had recommended it, and I had wanted to find the opportunity to read it for some time. I had *nothing* but opportunity right now. I took the book from the table next to my bed and opened it; out fell the diagram of my heart that my mother had showed me on Tuesday after my angiogram. She had folded it and placed it in my book for safekeeping. I unfolded the paper and studied it very intently for a great length of time. This was *my* heart … the internal metronome that beats in time to keep me alive, but it looked to be in such dismal, pathetic shape now.

I looked at all the areas that now had stents. I saw the numbers that translated into the percentages of blockages. I saw the areas that had smaller blockages, that may need addressing somewhere down the road. I had seen it that day in CCU, but as I studied it keenly, it was as if everything was finally hitting me. *This* was my heart now! *This* was my new reality. My future life was that of a heart patient. When I poured over it, I realized just how many areas had been affected and I also realized just how close I came. It could have easily gone the other way. All those things that I had anxiously worried over the night before my first angiogram *could* have come true.

I broke down in tears. With all I had been through, I think that this was the first time that I had really cried. I think that perhaps I was just too afraid to cry earlier. This cry was not just a little distressed cry. This was a completely *devastated, sobbing, gut wrenching, downright broken-hearted cry*. This was the cry that Oprah referred to as "the ugly cry." You know the kind that you cry when you just cannot control the convulsive, sighing reflex in your chest and you utter short gasping breaths? I was weeping uncontrollably, and I had a feeling of foreboding that I could not shake. I was telling myself, "This can't be good for your heart, what if you bring on another heart attack?" I just *could not* stop though. This went on for a while and very gradually as time passed, it went from outright inconsolable, uncontrollable weeping—to a sniveling whimper.

I felt so abandoned by the hospital staff too. After all, I *was* wearing a heart monitor. Surely I thought, with that little melt down something must have registered on their monitor. Wouldn't they have seen some sort of blips or *something* with such a poignant outburst? But, no one came in to check on me. I thought, "I could die down here all by myself and no one would know." That was *not* a comforting thought. That added to my night of increasing distress.

Where was that strong Cajun woman in these moments? Were these stents now my Kryptonite? Were my heart related issues now going to define me? I was sorry that I had *pretended* to be so brave and had sent my family home, but I knew that they needed their rest, too. I just wanted, no I *needed*, someone to talk to, a friendly voice to bring me comfort. It was now about 11:30 p.m. and I figured that all my family was in bed; at least I hoped that they were. I got my cell phone out and started looking through my list of contacts. I was looking for someone that I could call who would be awake at this time, and who wouldn't think that I was totally nuts. Sadly, not many people on my list of contacts met that criteria. There were two people that I *nearly* called, but I changed my mind. I was afraid they might think that I had lost it, and call my family and wake them up.

I had sat up on the side of my bed. I needed to use the restroom. I was getting ready to buzz the nurse for assistance. This was going to be my first time getting up in several days. I wanted to be sure that I wasn't weak or dizzy; I didn't need to fall. About that time, my nurse popped in to check on me. He helped me walk to the restroom and waited outside for me, he then helped me back to bed. He apparently sensed that I was distressed because he sat down at the foot of my bed and talked with me for some time. I found out during our conversation that he was a smoker. I scolded him about that. As a friend's dad used to say, "Why buy trouble, you're going to get enough for free." I told him he needed to quit that bad habit, look what had happened to me and I had never even smoked.

I told him that I had been concerned earlier because I could hear a lot of shouting off and on. I asked him if he knew what the problem was. I told him that it sounded like it was coming from the room next door. He laughed and told me yes, he knew exactly to what I was referring. He said that I heard *him* shouting. He explained that the patient next door to me was hard of hearing and he had to shout in order for the man to be able to hear him. He apologized for the noise. Boy, did I feel *silly* for overreacting.

I asked him if he was sure that my heart monitor was actually connected at the nurse's station and he assured me that it was. I told him about my little melt down. He told me that evidently, my heart rhythm had not gone into any arrhythmias or the monitor would have picked that up. I wasn't altogether sure if that was the case.

I did feel better just having someone to talk with, someone who had a clue as to what I was feeling. I know I couldn't have been the first of his patients to feel this way. I guess too, I was just feeling sorry for myself. I was having my own little "pity party" all by myself, but I needed to stop that now. Tomorrow was a new day and I hoped that the worst was behind me, I thought, "From here on out, I just need to focus on getting better." To use a quote that my cousin used to tell her son, I needed to "toughen-up bud."

It was then after midnight and my nurse suggested that I might be able to relax if I would take a sleeping pill. Normally when I am at home the only thing that I'll take to help me sleep is sinus medicine. I only take this rarely and I cannot take it late at night, or I will still be feeling its effects when I awake in the morning. This isn't good especially if I have to be somewhere early in the morning. Therefore, if I do take something, I would take it no later than 9:00 p.m. Since it was then well after midnight, out of habit, I told him that I couldn't take a sleeping pill so late at night because I would be hung over in the morning.

He looked at me, smiled, and said, "Where do you have to be in the morning? You won't be driving will you?"

I smiled back and said, "You've got a point; it's probably what I need."

He brought the sleeping pill and it did help to relax me. I was finally able to drift off and get some *much-needed* rest.

When I think back on that night, I do think the release of emotion that I felt when I broke down, was sorely needed. I feel it was probably cathartic for me because sometimes a "good cry" can be beneficial for women. It was good for me to be alone that night too. If someone had stayed with me that night, I wouldn't have gotten "all that" out of my system. Tomorrow was to be a new day with new twists to the saga.

CHAPTER 18

Friday, August 19, 2011

Morning had *finally* come ... at last. I awoke feeling better than I had the night before. Although, I think that it probably would have been impossible to feel any worse. As previously stated, the day starts early in a hospital. (I know I keep stating the obvious. You may have figured out by now, that I'm *not* a morning person.) In a hospital there is always a lot of activity taking place. There were medical personnel in and out taking my temperature and blood pressure. My blood sugar as well was checked several times a day. Considering everything in recent days, it had been on-track so far. That was a good thing because I knew that when you're under a lot of stress, your blood sugar could be adversely affected.

Was this day perhaps the day that I would be going home? I *longed* to be back at home in my own bed. After inquiring, I learned that you're never discharged directly from CCU; you must spend some time in a regular room first, so that you can be observed. *I* felt I had met that criteria and personally didn't see any reason why I needed to stay longer. My procedures were over and had been successful. My IV port was still in my arm, but wasn't connected to fluids any longer. *I* felt that I could do at home, exactly what I was doing there, which was just lying around, taking it easy. I just wanted to *go home*!

My mother arrived early; she wanted to be there when my doctor made his rounds. My breakfast was delivered and I was able to eat some of it, but I still didn't have much of an appetite. Next, a doctor and nurse practitioner came in to talk to me. This wasn't the cardiologist who had performed my procedures; it was his colleague from the cardiology group. He relayed to me that he was taking Dr. Nair's place since he had left for a trip to India that morning, and would be gone for the next few weeks. I didn't really like hearing that since Dr. Nair was the one who was familiar with my case; he *literally* knew my heart inside and out. On the other hand, I knew of this doctor's reputation and it was a good one. I knew though, my doctor deserved some time off from all the stressful work that he does, so I accepted this change reasonably well.

I had convinced *myself* that I would probably go home today, but then again, the doctor had other ideas. He said that I needed to stay a little longer and that was *not* what I wanted to hear. I felt irritated with him because I *just* wanted to go home. The next thing he told me was even more unpleasant. In my mind, I thought the worst was over now. I knew that my procedures had been successful; the blockages that had caused my heart attack were open now. *I* figured that all I needed to do was to go home to rest and recover. *I* thought that it was just a matter of taking good care of myself, this along with the passage of time would help me to get stronger and get better.

The doctor's next revelation would shock me completely; he said that I would need to be reevaluated in about three months for an implantable cardioverter defibrillator (ICD) and/ or a pacemaker. Here I was thinking that I was over the hump, starting on the home stretch toward recovery, this news made me wonder if I was even in the race at all. An ICD is a small, electronic device inserted under the skin, near the heart that continually monitors the rhythm of the heart. If it senses an abnormal rhythm or arrhythmia, it will deliver an electric shock to restore a normal rhythm. I didn't want surgery, *much less* a device *implanted* in my chest that could shock me! I was completely *stunned* by this news! Too surprised to even think to ask the reason *why* I might need this device. He let me know that they were still trying to get my new medications regulated as well. I didn't know it thus far, but there was yet *another shoe to fall* the *next* morning. I think doctors try to keep you on a need-to-know basis. I guess breaking things to you gradually is better than dumping it all on you at once.

I was so disappointed that I couldn't go home. I told my mother after the doctor left, that *all* I wanted was to go home so that I could get a real bath and wash my hair. This was Friday and my last authentic bath and head washing had been on Monday night, so my mother offered to help me to get a shower. This went fairly well, but I found it necessary to sit down in the shower chair, because after just a short time, I felt weak and tired. Was *this* what my new life was going to be like? That thought made me feel even more depressed. My mother helped me wash my hair, and dried it for me, it looked horrible but at least it smelled better. Having clean hair usually makes a girl feel better, and I guess it helped a bit.

I was now *exhausted* from all the exertion and I got back into bed to rest. While resting I watched the news and weather; there was a tropical storm out in the Atlantic, tropical storm Irene. When you live in South Louisiana as we do, weather is something that warrants monitoring. We *must* be watchful for changes or new developments. Being raised in this area, it's just something that we have become accustomed to doing. We *don't* like it, but it's an accepted part of living here. Over the years, we've weathered many storms; the most recent major storms were hurricanes Katrina and Gustav.

Preparing for a significant storm is long, *hard* work and this is the case whether you stay or you evacuate. First, *everything* in your yard has to be secured. You have to put plywood up over all the windows and doors. You have to buy extra gasoline, shop for food, batteries, and other necessities. You have to make sure that you have an ample supply of your medications, make arrangements for the pets, and pack up clothes and things that cannot be replaced, as well as, gather together all of your important papers. This was just the *short* list of a few things that needed to be done. My husband and I usually work as a team to get it all accomplished, and it's *still* hard work.

At that time, all I could anxiously think was, "We don't need this storm to come our way." Since I felt so weak and fragile there would have been *no way* I could have done all that was necessary if it did come in our direction. In reality, I couldn't do *anything* right now and besides that, I was still *stuck* here in this hospital bed. I remember thinking, "I hope that it goes in another direction," except, I couldn't help but thinking about others. I dejectedly thought, "No matter where this thing goes, there are other people in the same situation that I'm in and who feel just like I do, right now. They don't need this either." I felt guilty for wishing it in another direction. It was something new about which to be concerned. It would prove to be a non-issue for South Louisiana, but I didn't know that at the time.

The eventual outcome was that Irene did become the first major hurricane of the 2011 season. It became a category 3 storm and made landfall, first on the outer banks of North Carolina, continuing up the east coast making its final landfall in Brooklyn, New York.

As the day wore on, I had numerous phone calls from concerned friends and family, so many people wanted to check on me. I started to get visitors, as well and there was a constant stream of people coming and going all day. I've tried to remember everyone who came by that day, I may have forgotten some, but there were at least twenty-five visitors, if not more. By the end of the day, I felt *totally exhausted.* I most likely had *way* too much company that day, but I felt in a way, renewed and encouraged by the love and kindness of so many who were pulling for me to get better.

I felt *so* tired that I could hardly keep my eyes open. The way I felt then, I didn't think that I would need a sleeping pill that night. My younger daughter had opted to spend the night with me. She was working the next day there at the hospital, but said she really wanted to stay. I *didn't* resist, I had learned my lesson the night before. She settled in on the little sofa that makes into a bed that was in my room and we both fell sound asleep.

Some time during the middle of the night, my nurse awakened me.

He was gently shaking me and saying, "Ms. Kim, are you okay."

I was in a deep sleep at the time; I opened my eyes and said, "Yes, I think so. Why?"

He told me that he noticed that my blood pressure had dropped while I was sleeping. He said my bottom number was at 35, so he just wanted to make sure that I was okay. I reassured him that I felt fine. I got up and went to the restroom and my numbers improved. He then told me that my blood pressure medication was the one that they were still trying to regulate. That now made sense and the dosage *evidently* needed to be adjusted once more. I deduced that the doctor was right again when he wanted me to stay an extra day. Had I gone home, I would have never realized that there was an issue with my blood pressure while sleeping. This episode also proved to me that they actually *were* monitoring me at the nurse's station. I remembered having serious doubts about that the night before.

CHAPTER 19

Saturday, August 20, 2011

I awoke to a bright, sunny morning and was encouraged that it was going to be a good day. I had been able to get some much-needed rest last night and was optimistically anticipating that it would be the day I would be able to go home. My husband didn't have to work that day, so he came to the hospital early that morning, he was also thinking I would be released today. It's just so difficult when a family member is in the hospital; life simply can't get back to normal until your loved one comes home.

I had just finished my breakfast when the doctor made his rounds. If you will remember, I said that there was yet another shoe to fall. Well, if I were to use a colloquial reference, it was more of a large, white shrimp boot. The doctor came in, and in a quick, concise manner told me that I could be discharged, but I couldn't go home until I was fitted with device called a Life Preserver*. I thought, "A life preserver, what is that?" It sounded like something that you would wear on a boat.

*name changed

He said that someone was coming from out of town to fit me with it and to teach me how to operate it. *And* that I would have to wear it for the next three months, until I could be reevaluated to determine if the implantable defibrillator was necessary. I was completely *stunned*, *confused*, and *speechless*, and that doesn't happen very often. As you have probably figured out by now, I am reasonably efficient at asking questions, but I didn't even know *what* to ask. He didn't really go into many details; at least I don't *think* that he did. I was so taken aback that I wasn't actually sure. He may have thought that the cardiologist who had performed my procedures had explained things to me, but he hadn't, and he was now out of the country. The doctor had now left my room. My husband and I just stared at each other with our eyes wide and mouths open.

I blurted out, "*What* was that all about? A *life preserver?* ... **THREE MONTHS?**"

I had been waiting to hear that I could go home, but this was much more than I had bargained for. I *really* didn't understand the whys and wherefores of what had just happened.

But, the very next person who came into my room though, I *did* have questions for them and for the *next* person after that. The problem was that no one really knew a lot about it and I was getting nothing but vague answers. What was this thing? Where was this mystery person coming from? When would they get here? No one knew. This was important to me, because the doctor had said that I *could not leave*, until *It*, whatever *It* was, had arrived. I talked to my family about it and they were as confused as I was. I finally came to the conclusion that I had figured out the reason. I said, "They must have checked out my insurance and this is probably just something that they can bill the insurance company for. It can't be *that* serious." I knew by this time that my insurance was probably paying at 100%.

At long last, a nurse came in who did have a few answers. I wanted to know why I needed this and she was finally able to give me a tangible answer. Of course, I didn't really understand what she was talking about at the time. She said that I needed this device because I had a low ejection fraction, which was just under 20%. She said that it was *now* the standard of care to send patients home with this device when their ejection fraction was below 35%. At the time, I thought that she was saying "injection fraction," ... and I didn't know what *either* were.

I asked why no one seemed to know much about it. She said that it wasn't new, but that it was *newly* in use in this area. She told me that it wasn't necessary for the majority of patients and she had only known three patients to go home with the device. OH, GREAT! I needed this new device that no one knew anything about, and only a few people required, leave it to me to need something out of the ordinary.

I looked directly into her eyes and said, "Am I really *that* bad off that I need this?"

I guess I put her on the spot because she paused, smiled kindly and tried to soften her answer by saying, "It's *just* a precaution for your protection."

I was less than thrilled, to say the least. I still didn't have the big picture yet, but I certainly did not like what was coming into focus.

I would see more pieces of the picture a few days later, after I finally went home. This was when my friend and her daughter, who is a nurse, came to visit then. She explained ejection fraction to me in terms, which I, as a non-professional, could grasp. This was what I learned an ejection fraction to be. She said it's a measure of the amount of blood your heart pumps or ejects out of a filled pumping chamber with each heartbeat. It's the sum of blood pumped out divided by the entire amount of blood in a filled ventricle. It's usually measured on the left ventricle, the principal pumping chamber of the heart. It's used to detect and monitor heart failure by determining how well the heart is functioning. Normal is anywhere from 50% to 60%, mine was less than 20%. I had no idea at the time just how serious this could be. This probably was a good thing, perhaps that's why the doctor may not have elaborated.

I would learn the full picture a week later when I went for my check-up with the cardiologist. These percentages were determined when I had the echocardiogram in CCU. With a low ejection fraction, blood is allowed to sit still longer inside the heart. Blood that isn't moving is more likely to form clots, which can in turn cause cardiac arrest or put you at risk for a stroke. I would also learn that with a low ejection fraction there is an increased risk for dangerous arrhythmias of the heart. Even though I didn't fully understand at the time, I was sensing that what I was dealing with was serious. This was a *total surprise* to me, because as I had said earlier, I was thinking that everything was going to be fine since my procedures had all gone well. I thought that my heart was pretty much *"fixed."* I thought I just needed to go home and finish the healing process. I didn't realize that I still had a very, very long way to go.

While waiting for this person to arrive with this Life Preserver, my daughter came up to my room on her break to check on me. We told her about what had been going on. She took out her phone and pulled up "Life Preserver." It showed a picture of the device. It looked like something a terrorist would wear; it had wires and sensors all around. It also had these three large metallic pads, one in the front and two in the back. She started reading about it. It was a *wearable, automated, external, defibrillator*. Wonderful! Just what I've always wanted, my very own electric undergarment.

We were still waiting, but in the meantime, I did have a few visitors that day. It wasn't as many as the day before, *but* that was okay. I now had a lot on my mind to deal with. As I think back now, the time delay was most likely a good thing because it gave me more time to adjust to the idea of this new, *unwelcome* development.

My daughter had been invited to her cousin's graduation party that night and she told me she didn't think she was going to go. It was a theme party—"Sequins and Sneakers." Everyone was going to wear semi-formal clothing and high top sneakers, it sounded like a fun, clever idea. She already had her outfit for the party so I insisted that she go. I felt that she wanted to stay home on my account; I sensed she felt guilty about leaving me and I didn't want that. I supposed she thought the people at the party would think badly of her since her mom was in the hospital while she was out partying and dancing. However, I knew that she needed a break from all this hospital stuff. She had been so helpful and devoted, but she's young and needed to be with young, fun, happy people. I refused to take "no" for an answer and told her that I would be upset if she didn't go. I told my older daughter, who is a hairdresser, to take her sister home and make her *gorgeous*. She was going to that party if I had anything to say about it. My only request was for her to take plenty of pictures. I also asked her to stop by the hospital after the party was over so that I could see her in her dress. It took some convincing, but she finally agreed to go.

CHAPTER 20

One bright spot in my day was a nurse's assistant who had been taking care of me since I had been transferred to a regular room. She had such a pleasant, amusing nature, with personality plus. She was, in essence, a ray of sunshine in such a gloomy place and I actually enjoyed her visits. I asked her if she thought there would be any chance that I would be able to go home once this mystery person would come. She said that I couldn't leave until the doctor issued my discharge papers and since it was late in the day on a Saturday afternoon, it seemed *unlikely* today. I had figured as much, but I was still hopeful.

About 5:00 p.m. the person that my husband and I had waited on *all day*, had finally arrived. She was a cardiac nurse and had driven down from Baton Rouge, which is about two hours away from where we live. She apologized for coming so late and explained that she had to work a health fair earlier in the day. She then began to explain to us how the unit worked. She told us that the device continuously monitors your heart. If it detected a life-threatening rhythm, the device would then deliver a "treatment" to restore a normal rhythm. The "treatment" was an electrical shock and in a satirical way, it was humorous, how she kept saying "treatment" instead of shock. I guess it was to diminish the fright value so that it didn't sound as threatening.

The unit consisted of several different components. She needed to measure me for the first component, called the garment; it was the cloth portion that you wore. It had an electrode belt attached to it and was to be worn under your clothing, *touching* your skin. The four electrodes around the belt were what monitored your heartbeat. Three defibrillator pads fit into the garment and these were what actually delivered the "treatment."

In the center back of the garment was a vibration box, but I'll tell more about that, later. She measured me to be sure that it was the proper fit, it needed to be snug, but not tight. I asked if I would be able to wear a bra with it. She said yes, but it had to be worn on top of the garment. In addition, the bra couldn't be an underwire bra; this was to prevent burns in the event that a "treatment" was delivered. That did make sense.

The next component was the monitor. It fit inside a holster with an adjustable neck strap that made it look like a large camera. It also had a red light on the front that blinked once per second. This was the main computerized unit of the system and it monitored your heartbeat through the electrode belt, connected by a small cable. If it sensed an abnormal rhythm (or no rhythm at all) it delivered a shock treatment (or as the manual put it "defibrillating energy") by means of the metallic defibrillator pads. There were two defibrillator pads in the back and one in the front, just below the left breast. The monitor had a touch-screen that displayed different messages about how the device operated, allowing you to interact with the device. There was a menu button where you could select different options, you could, for instance, check the battery level. It came with two batteries so that you could always have one in the device and one recharging. There was also a help screen if you encountered any problems operating the unit (I felt sure that I would need to use that option, *often*).

The last component was the charger unit, which recharged the battery and communicated wirelessly with the monitor. By means of the charger unit, at the end of each day, all the data recorded throughout that day was automatically uploaded to the company that manufactured the device. They, in turn, would transmit the data to my doctor for review.

Whew! That was a lot of information for me to process. I had trouble programming my cell phone or a VCR, how in the world was I going to be able to operate this thing? Here I was, *electronically challenged*, wearing a state-of-the-art device worth thousands of dollars—that could shock me. I felt so overwhelmed and dismayed. At least my husband was with me for this crash course, but I sensed that he was overwhelmed too.

She showed us how to assemble all the parts in the garment. It was color coded, but could be a little tricky. She put the unit on me and recorded my heartbeat. She told me to *never* let anyone try it on; she said if someone else would wear it, the unit wouldn't recognize *their* heartbeat and would then process it as an abnormal rhythm. It would then deliver a "treatment." *Wow !*

She stressed that it could only protect me if I was wearing it and that meant that I would *only* be allowed to take it off for a short bath and by no means should it get wet. There was *so much* to remember and I worried that I would forget something *important*. Thankfully, there was a manual to refer to and a twenty-four hour a day help line and she encouraged me *not* to hesitate to call with any issue that I had. I was somewhat relieved that help would only be a phone call away.

There was still more that I needed to learn though. She explained that there were different types of alarms. There was a gong alert, this low-pitched, gong-type sound repeated once every second. This signal indicated that there was a minor problem that needed addressing. It may *gong* if there was a problem, for instance, with the belt not being fastened properly or one of the electrodes not making proper contact with the skin. This one was no big deal; it just required a little attention.

There was a vibration alert from the vibration box located in the center of my back, that I referred to earlier. You would get a vibration alert immediately before you were about to get a siren alert. Now the *siren alert* was a high-pitched, multi-tone alert that meant an abnormal rhythm had been detected. There were two buttons (the response buttons) that must be simultaneously pressed in order to stop the treatment from being delivered. *If* these buttons were *not* pressed when you heard the siren alarm, you would receive a treatment within one minute. This one *was* a big deal.

I was instructed with a siren alarm, as long as I was able—I was to continue to press the response buttons. She said with a siren alarm, I was to sit or lie down, because there was good chance that I could become unconscious. She told us, *no one else* was to press the response buttons, only the patient. I wanted to know what if I really needed a treatment and was stopping it from occurring by pressing these buttons. She said if a treatment was necessary, that I would ultimately pass out and with no one pressing the buttons, a treatment would then be delivered. Next, a voice prompt would instruct bystanders not to touch me and to call for an ambulance. She warned my husband if a siren alarm would go off in the middle of the night and I was unconscious, unable to press the buttons, *do not* touch me. She told him that he could be in bed next to me, but if he were touching me at the time a treatment was administered, he would be shocked as well. I was afraid he wouldn't want to sleep next to me once we went home. (After the fact, he told me that this *had been* a serious concern to him for all those months that I had to wear the device.) In addition, she gave us instructions as to what to do in the event that I actually did receive a treatment.

Upon learning all of this, now I *really* did feel like I was being fitted with a bomb. I knew its purpose, but I didn't like the idea one bit. How was I going to wear this for three months? She next started to give me instructions on how to put the unit into airplane mode. "*WHAT?*" I told her I didn't need any instruction on that because there was *no way* I was getting on a plane wearing that thing. You couldn't get on a plane with a pair of embroidery scissors without someone going ballistic, much less something like this. That would have been all I needed, to have airport security think I was a terrorist wearing a bomb. She said occasionally there could be a death in the family and a person may then have to fly.

I told her, "I don't care who dies, I'm *not* getting on an airplane with *that thing*!" and I meant it too!

She told me refer to my manual often. In fact, she recommended that I read it from cover to cover when I got home. That sounded like a very good idea because she had showed and told me *a lot* in a short span of time. She shared with me several other tips that I might need, but then needed to leave to go back home. I was so unsure if I would retain everything that she had taught me. I hoped that I would remember, but feared I wouldn't because it was *plenty* to process, and quite overwhelming. Here I was now wearing this *thing* that was supposed to protect me and save my life, and I feared that it was going to give me another heart attack. I felt tremendously frazzled now.

I felt so depressed too. I had no idea that I even needed something like this. I knew that a heart attack is a serious thing, but to have a doctor tell you that you cannot go home without this device, he's saying that your life may depend on it. I felt weak, and weary, and strained. I felt like I was *crumpled* ... *crumpled* deep within my soul, just like a piece of paper. Once a piece of paper is crumpled, you can never get the wrinkles out, no matter how hard that you try. That was how I felt on the inside. I thought that I would never be the same—never whole again.

My husband was going to stay with me that night. This was the first time in five days that my husband and I had been alone to actually talk seriously. I started pouring out my innermost fears and feelings to him. With a sigh of anguish, I told him, "My life, as I *knew* it ... is over. I'll never be the same. I'll just be this pathetic person from here on out."

If you'll remember, that was one of my concerns my first night in CCU. I had heard the term "cardiac cripple." Was that what I was now? I told him I *hated* that this had happened and that I didn't want to be a burden to him. Feeling so *frail* and *useless* as I did, I knew that I would have to depend on him and my girls now.

He tenderly looked at me and in a soft, reassuring tone said, "It doesn't matter. You're here with me, that's all that counts, no matter what happens. As for you being a burden, *don't* think like that. Even if I have to help you, that's okay, as long as I have you by my side. You know what *would* have been a burden? If I had lost you and had to go through my life without you, *that* would have been a burden, not this."

The love and compassion was evident in his voice. These words were so touching to hear and I knew that he meant every word of it. It did make me feel better just hearing it and certainly gave me an adjustment to my thinking. He also reminded me about my father. He wanted me to recall *all* that my father had been through, and to think of how well he had recovered. My father is like the Energizer Bunny, he just keeps on going. My husband told me if my father could have such a good outcome, then I could too. I *so* hoped that he was right.

The first chapter of this saga was behind us now. The next chapter in our lives was just ahead. All that night, he lovingly gazed at me with his sweet smile, but his dark blue eyes could not hide the worry that he was trying to keep inside. We didn't know exactly what was ahead for us, but we were going to face it together, as a couple. We had vowed a *long* time ago, in sickness and in health, forever and always …

As we sat talking and watching television together, we even held hands. These moments between us felt like we were back to our teen years as high school sweethearts. We were transported back to the time when our love was new. These events of late had intensified the already strong bond between us. This was the first *normal* time between us in a week. We really did need that time together to reconnect. We even went on a date "of sorts." We went for a walk down to the nurse's station, just the three of us, my husband, *my bomb,* and me. That was another first, my first walk in a week. It was a slow walk but it was *steps* in the right direction.

When we got down to the nurse's station, I spotted a scale. I told my husband that I wondered if I had lost any weight. I definitely had not been eating much. I had him hold the monitor part of my device. I stepped on the scale and was surprised to see that I had lost seven pounds that week. I was delighted; I had never lost that much in such a short time. As I said earlier, weight loss had never come easily for me.

The nurse at the desk smiled, and said, "She must be getting better. When a woman starts to worry about her weight again, that means she is on the mend."

I sure hoped that was the case and I was going to try my best to watch my diet in hopes of losing my excess weight. I knew now, that was more important than ever for my health. We slowly walked back to my room at the end of the hall. I felt tired after my little walk and I got back in bed to rest.

About 10 p.m., my daughter came to see me as she had promised she would. She looked *absolutely beautiful* in her party dress; her sister had done a stunning job on her hair and makeup. I was so glad she had agreed to go to the party since I knew how much she needed a break. She was exhausted from her stressful week, so she didn't stay out late. She had also brought us a piece of cake, I ate just two small bites, and that was it. Surprisingly, I was okay with that little taste; I hoped that I had turned over a new leaf with my eating habits. She went home and we settled in for the night. I was still very uncomfortable and ill at ease with my new device, being on edge that it would shock me at any moment. I slept *very lightly*, on and off all during the night.

CHAPTER 21

Sunday morning, August 21, 2011

Perhaps I could now go home and trusted there was *nothing else* that would prevent that from happening today. I didn't want any more shoes (or boots) to fall. A new cardiologist came around this morning and he said the magic words I had longed to hear—

"We are going to discharge you this morning. You can go home."

Finally! I was getting to go home. Of course, everything must be processed through channels, things don't happen immediately at a hospital, with the exception of the emergency room ... *maybe*? The nurse assistant, that I had become fond of, warned us it might take a little while and she encouraged us to try to relax while waiting.

She later brought in my discharge papers, a packet of eighteen different papers. These instructions stated that I needed to go back for a follow-up visit with the cardiologist in a week. It also contained a list of my diagnoses, procedures performed, a follow-up plan, activity limitations and detailed instructions on how to care for myself, once I went home. In addition, there was the list of medications prescribed, how and when to take them, along with a handful of scripts to have filled at the pharmacy. Besides my manual for my device, I now needed to read these too and wanted to do this as soon as possible so I could make sure I wasn't missing something important. Okay, here again, there was a lot of information to process, but I was going to give it my best.

Finally, the moment had arrived and I couldn't have been more thrilled. The nurse assistant wheeled me out to my car, gave me a big hug and wished me well. I don't know who was happier, my husband or me. It was almost lunchtime, so I had my husband pick up a salad for me on the way home. We next went by the pharmacy to drop off the stack of scripts to have filled. We didn't want to wait, so we said someone would come back for them. The next stop was *home*.

When we got there my daughters, son-in-law and grandson were there to meet us; it felt so good to be back home with my family. My grandson was fascinated with Mawsie's new "fashion accessory" (my bomb). My older daughter had been stressing over getting the house clean and ready for my homecoming. She knows that I am a particular person and the housework had gone by the way side for the two weeks preceding the heart attack. I had been in so much pain that I had let so much slide. Besides that, my being in the hospital for a week with my family in and out of the house during that time, to say the least, it *needed* some attention.

My daughter said cleaning house for me felt like cleaning for a combination of Martha Stewart and Hitler. I *really* hoped that she was exaggerating. She was worried it wouldn't be up to my standards. My girls teased me, calling me "Martha Hitler." I told them that everything looked fine; I was just relieved to be home again and that I really did appreciate all their hard work and help. They would continue to help me where they could, in the days to come. I ate my salad and then needed to rest. It was as if I'd done a day's work; it sure didn't take much for me to become tired now. I wanted a "real" bath, but I *needed* a nap more. I was able to nap in my own bed, as I snuggled down in the cool, crisp, softly scented sheets, it felt so wonderful. I *had* missed it so!

After my nap, my younger daughter came home from the pharmacy with my new medications and dumped them all out on the kitchen counter. There were eight medication bottles, all with *different* instructions. I definitely wasn't ready for this new challenge. I had been taking these medicines in the hospital and had received some of them that morning according to my discharge papers, but I needed to decipher which ones. I needed to do this right because this was of utmost importance. Everyone at the hospital had told me, "Take your medications—*that* is what is going to heal your heart." Again, I was overwhelmed. My daughter thankfully had the presence of mind to purchase a medicine caddy as well, the type that divides the medication for different times of the day. The one that I used to think, were for "old people" to use, I guess I was now officially an "old person," and I *had* the medicine caddy to prove it. It sure felt like I had aged in the last week.

One of my good friends had stopped by to bring us food for supper since I wouldn't be cooking right away. Cajun people are very good about things like that.

Characteristically, Cajun's are known for being generous, hospitable, caring people. They know how to take care of you without you even needing to ask for help. This close friend is a very meticulous, organized person. She could see how distressed I was over this medicine dilemma, so she took control. She reviewed my list from the hospital that showed everything I had taken so far that day, organized it all, and wrote out a detailed list of what I needed to take and when. She even marked the bottles with the times that I should take them. I was so grateful that she did this; she relieved me of a giant stress. These are the little things that can be so stressful that most people don't even think about *until* faced with them. Normally, I was in the role of the caregiver, but when the caregiver is also the patient, this can make the lines a little more blurred ... and challenging.

My older daughter reminded me that I *had* to get better because we all had plans for November. Every fall she takes her dad to a Saints football game at the Superdome, it was just a yearly, father/daughter thing. While they are at the football game, my thoughtful son-in-law takes my younger daughter and me to lunch and then shopping. He takes us to historic Magazine Street; it's six miles long and filled with the most fabulous little antique shops, restaurants, and art galleries imaginable. We always have a great time. I do have a very special son-in-law that will do that for his mother-in-law and I'm appreciative of this fact. As much as I enjoy this yearly outing, I couldn't even think that far ahead. I told her I would just have to wait to see how things were by then. I couldn't make those plans that far in advance, at least not right now.

Next, I was going to get that longed-for bath. All I needed to do was to remember how to take this device off correctly since this would be the first time I would do that on my own. I disconnected the cable from the monitor and it started to *"GONG." Just great!* I couldn't remember what I had done wrong; I just knew that it wasn't right! My friend was still visiting, so I sent the monitor out to her, still "gonging," with instructions to get the manual out to try to figure out what I had done wrong. At least I knew it couldn't shock me because the cable wasn't connected. Here I was, becoming all worked up over this and my device was off, so I wasn't protected. Again, *just great!* My daughter helped me get my bath and wash my hair. It was not the relaxing bath that I had envisioned, but it was definitely better than *any* bath that I had while in the hospital. I tried to be quick so that I would not be *unprotected* for long.

Now, I would have to put it all back on. My friend had figured out that I was supposed to take the battery out *first* before disconnecting the cable. Yes, now I remembered, it didn't have an on/off switch; you had to disconnect the battery first. I fumbled through the process, but *finally* got it all on correctly. Again, I was *exhausted* from all that work.

My daughter, the hairdresser, dried and styled my hair for me. It was the best it had looked all week, maybe even the last three weeks. My parents came over to visit for a while. I joked with my father; I told him if he had to give me an *inheritance*, I would have preferred stocks, bonds or cash instead of the *legacy* of heart disease. We all visited and just enjoyed being together until my daughter and son-in-law had to leave to go back to New

Orleans. It had been a long day, but I was finally home, and that made me happy.

Now, I felt I could officially start my recovery process and we could resume our lives once again. My family decided that I should not be alone at first, in case I needed help. My family and friends had all picked a day for that week and they were going to come to "babysit" me. I hated to take them away from their regular routines, but I was glad they had volunteered to stay with me; it made me feel more secure. When I was with people, I had less time to think and stress over my own issues.

CHAPTER 22

It had been a long day; it had been a long, whirlwind week for that matter. We were worn-out, so we went to bed early; greatly needing some sleep after all we had been through in the last week. My husband had to return to work in the morning. I could tell by his breathing that he fell asleep right away. I just wished I could as well. Again, the room was dark and quiet. Was this going to be a fitful night with some resemblance to my first night in CCU? Like that night, my thoughts were dark, and my restless mind again, was *far* from quiet.

I pondered deeply over the events from that long week. I wondered what lay ahead for me. At this point, I still didn't understand the whole ejection fraction thing very well, but I had deduced that it had to be something serious. After all, it was the reason I was wearing this device. The woman, who fitted me with it, had told me, as the electrodes monitored my heart, there were specifically, two abnormal rhythms that would cause it to deliver a treatment. They were ventricular fibrillation and ventricular tachycardia. It would deliver a treatment in the event that my heart would stop beating as well. I had read in the manual that both of these abnormal rhythms, if left untreated, could lead to cardiac arrest, which is usually followed by sudden cardiac death. I was no "rocket surgeon" but I was smart enough to put two and two together. Whatever this ejection fraction thing was, it put me at risk for a possibly fatal cardiac event. That realization, along with the fact that I was feeling much more emotional now, was not conducive to getting a good night sleep.

I was even second-guessing myself for being in such a hurry to want to go home from the hospital. I had longed to be home. Then again, at least when I was in the hospital, if I needed help it was nearby. I lived twenty minutes away from the hospital; what if I needed help right away? On the other hand, I knew I couldn't stay at the hospital indefinitely and besides that, I had no choice *now*. As I lay there in the quiet stillness of night, I felt very aware of my heartbeat, which was good *and* bad. Good, in that it was still beating keeping me alive. It was bad, in that every time it fluttered or twinged, I worried that something was going wrong.

Then of course, there is this little matter of the fact that I am wearing the equivalent of what I consider to be a *bomb*. It was most unsettling, I guess partly because it was something new that I had not yet accepted emotionally. I tried to reason with myself—"This thing is for my protection, it might save my life. It's really a good thing, but I'm so *afraid* to get shocked. What if it malfunctions? Devices malfunction all the time. What if I have the lemon in the bunch? It's supposed to shock me and restore a normal rhythm if I need it. What if it malfunctions and shocks me? My heart is already so pathetic, if it does, it'll kill me. Will it interpret that flutter or twinge I feel as abnormal and shock me? " This was just a brief sampling of my internal monologue that night.

Aside from the anxiety, there was the comfort issue. I normally slept on my left side. The monitor portion was on my right side, but with the strap around my neck connected to it, sleeping on my left side would be out of the question. I could have switched it to the left side, but then it would have been between my husband and I, and that wouldn't work either. If I turned on my right, then the monitor, being bulky and hard, was in my way. The only other option was to lie on my back, which I was not used to doing or comfortable in that position, but that seemed to be the best option. Since the defibrillator pads were directly touching my skin, I found that I perspired heavily where they rubbed. What's more, the vibration box pressed into my back. Then, there was the little matter of the red blinking light on the unit that blinked once every second. It was distracting and a constant reminder that it was there. This would take some getting used to, at the *very* least.

It was another *long, long* night for me. I nodded off a few times, but not for any extended period, I know this because I watched the clock much of the night. If I were to offer a guess, I would say that I *may* have slept a total of an hour all night, if that. I would soon come to see my bed in a whole new light. It would seem more like my enemy than my dear old friend.

CHAPTER 23

Monday, August 22, 2011

My husband got up at 5:00 a.m. for work. My friend who had organized my medication was going to be the first to "babysit" me and she was coming over about 8:00 a.m. My husband left shortly before 6:00 a.m., *I felt so alone*. After all, this was the first time in a week, since I had been truly on my own. I thought, "What if something happens to me before my friend gets here?" I felt afraid and I was also *exhausted* from lack of sleep. I tried to relax and sleep a little until she arrived. I did actually fall asleep, only to have a bad dream and I awoke frightened with my heart pounding like a drum. Was this going to cause my heart to go into an arrhythmia? Was this going to cause me to get a shock? I was disturbed and unnerved by the bad dream and wouldn't be able to get back to sleep. *Oh, how was I going to get better*? How was my heart going to heal if I couldn't get any rest? I was anxious for my friend to arrive. I tried to calm myself; I *didn't* want to be alone.

I thought at the hospital that going home was going to make me feel better. It did, in a way, but there were so many issues to deal with that I had not expected. Where was that woman of strong Cajun stock? Was she now a total basket case? I was trying to show strength on the outside to put my family's minds at ease because I didn't want them to worry excessively, but inside I felt like I was a total, wretched mess.

My friend arrived on time. I told her that I had a really bad night and asked if she would mind if I went back to bed, she encouraged me to get some rest. I did return to bed and was able to sleep until about noon, I felt somewhat better when I got up. I ate a light lunch and then decided to read over all the paperwork they had given me at the hospital when I was discharged.

These were the highlights:

I was to do **no heavy lifting, pulling, or pushing**. The doctor that had discharged me did tell me that he wanted me to walk in the house in order to get some moderate exercise; this would help me to get my strength back. There was a warning though to avoid *any* activity that would cause shortness of breath or chest pain.

I was to **monitor my weight,** by weighing first thing every morning and recording it. Any increase of two to three pounds over a few days needed to be reported to my doctor to be sure that excess fluid wasn't building up again. To assist with this, I was to *strictly* **limit my sodium** intake. I was to have no more than a total of 2000 mg. per day (since that time there has been a revision to the sodium limit. The limit per day is now 1500 mg.). That might sound like a generous amount, however almost everything you buy contains excessive amounts of sodium, and I would learn this was going to be a real challenge. I *had* been watching my sodium before, but now I needed to be even more careful. With my heart not functioning properly, excess sodium would make me retain more fluid, I couldn't handle any overindulgence. I was also to **monitor my blood pressure**, record the measurements and bring them to my next doctor appointment. So far, it had been on the low side of normal, which was where the doctor wanted it now, he said the lower the blood pressure, the less stress on the heart.

Another item discussed was to **eat a heart healthy diet,** low in saturated fat and cholesterol. I read through the suggestions of the diet plan, this was how we were eating already. At least this was one big change that I didn't have to *initiate*. I knew that this could be a huge hurdle for some who are abruptly faced with these major changes in diet. I had started to make some of those necessary changes years back; I would just have to be a little more careful now by being vigilant with portion control. I hoped to continue to lose more weight and so far, my appetite still hadn't come back, so that made it much easier. I was likewise to continue as before, watching my carb intake. I would later learn that I could have requested a dietitian to visit me while in the hospital; this would have assisted me with fine-tuning my diet. I wished that someone had told me I had that option while there.

The paper work stressed the importance of **taking medications properly** and this was something that I was determined to do. My friend's list was going to make that much easier to accomplish. I had been prescribed Nitroglycerine went I left the hospital; I was to carry it with me at all times and take as needed for chest pain. I remember as a young girl seeing my maternal grandfather taking nitroglycerin tablets. Those tiny pills that Pa Paw carried in that small, shiny, metal bottle intrigued me but I never thought that one day I would have to take them too. My grandfather had his heart attack in his early fifties, when I was six years old. That was the first time I had heard the word "angina." As a six year old, I recall thinking it was such a funny sounding word. In addition, my paper work recommended that I make a list of all my medications and carry it with me at all times. That was a good idea, because I knew I would never remember all of them.

There was also the recommendation to **reduce stress.** It said, "Stress causes an increased work load on the heart. Identifying stress reduction techniques that work for you are an important part of your recovery." The problem with that was, that my main stressor was going to be around my neck and strapped to my chest for the next three months. *So much for stress reduction, huh?*

The importance of **keeping appointments** with the cardiologists was also advised. At discharge, I was instructed to make my follow-up appointment for one week. I called and was given an appointment for the following Tuesday, August 30. As stated earlier, my cardiologist had gone out of the country, so I was scheduled to see Dr. Anil, the cardiologist that my husband and I had seen the night of the ABI screening. That screening had only taken place on July 26, it seemed so long ago, but not even a month had passed. So much had happened in such a short time. I also made another appointment for my daughter who had missed her appointment the day of my second angiogram.

As I read the paper work, I learned that the type of heart attack that I had, was called a Non-ST Elevation Myocardial Infarction (NSTEMI Heart Attack). It said, "This type of heart attack occurs when a blood vessel on the surface of the heart (coronary artery) is blocked and interrupts blood supply to the heart muscle. This blockage is usually caused by cholesterol buildup (atherosclerotic plaque) within a coronary artery. The plaque cracks which creates a rough surface where blood cells attach, forming a clot." I already knew that was *basically* what had occurred. The next thing I read, I did not know, and did not like. It said, "After an NSTEMI, there is a higher chance of another heart attack and returning angina after you have recovered." I fearfully thought, "A higher chance of *another* heart attack?" Oh no, I certainly didn't want that to happen.

"Returning angina?" Angina is chest pain or pressure that happens with exertion and goes away with rest. This is a warning that blood flow to the heart isn't enough. *That* was what had been occurring for the two weeks prior to my heart attack. According to what I was reading, I felt like I may still be a ticking time bomb, as well as the fact that I was wearing one.

That was some days work that I had done today, huh? At least I was doing it from my very own sofa instead of a hospital bed. I noticed that I got tired very quickly. I really enjoyed and appreciated my friend's visit; she kept me company until my husband came home. I was to have a new babysitter every day of that week.

I was so touched at the outpouring of love, kindness, and help showered on me. People responded in such varied and numerous ways—I received many phone calls, flowers, visits, and cards. There were so many who told me that they were keeping me in their prayers, *this* was most comforting and reassuring of all to me. Many friends and family cooked delicious meals for us. I know my husband and daughter appreciated that as much as I did since they were used to getting good home cooked meals. A good support system is so vital for a successful recovery; you just feel better knowing that others care about you.

Since my appetite wasn't what it should be, I tried to make every meal count. I felt confident that the healthier I ate; hopefully the faster I would heal. I had read— "food is medicine," so I tried to select only things that were the *most nutritious* for each meal and this was something that I would attempt to continue doing. I do think my stomach had shrunk though because I seemed to be full with much less food. One thing I did notice was that my tastes had changed. There were foods that I had eaten all my life, which *did not* appeal to me at all and I was baffled by this mystery. I don't know why, but cold foods seem to be more appealing to me than hot foods. I was eating mainly fresh fruit, yogurt, salad, hummus and whole-grain crackers.

I was still trying to get used to wearing my device. It wasn't only the thought of it, but also the physical part of actually wearing it too. It was on a long strap worn across my chest, and it hung at my right side. It weighed four pounds; try wearing a four-pound necklace all day, every day. It'll most definitely make your back and neck *ache*.

As I said earlier, I was only allowed to take it off for a bath and my husband really watched the clock while I was bathing. If he thought I was taking too long, he would remind me that it was time to get out and get my device back on. He made me promise that I wouldn't bathe unless someone was at home to monitor me.

It was necessary that the cloth portion be changed out every few days in order for it to be washed. This process was a bit daunting because all the wires on the sensors and defibrillator pads had to be put back just so in order for it to work properly. Thankfully, there was color-coding on the sensor belt, or I don't think we would have ever put it back together. My husband volunteered for this new job, he made the swap while I was in the tub so it could be ready to put on when I got out. My bath time limit was fifteen minutes, I enjoyed the feeling of freedom for that short time, but the idea that I was unprotected was ever present.

I remember wishing I could just go to sleep and wake up in three months. By then, the doctor felt they would know whether the reperfusion process had worked and I might know what my future held. The waiting game is excruciating and hard on the nerves, I just wanted to know what was going to happen to me. I guess patience is something that I need to *continue* to work on.

I tried to get back to doing normal things. I remember several days after getting out of the hospital; I decided to look through the newspaper. As I leafed through it, I came to the obituary page. It stirred in me a wave of emotion and I started to tear up, all I could think of was *my* picture and write-up could have been there. It was upsetting because it was a chilling reminder of what easily *could* have been.

A week had now passed since being discharged from the hospital. My family had finally consented to letting me stay by myself. I had "graduated," and was a big girl now. They did call throughout the day to check on me and yes, I was fine.

I decided to try to do something constructive with my time today. I had concerns about one of my closest friends who had always been so good to me (the same friend who had helped me with my bath in the hospital). She had several health issues that she wasn't making a priority in her life; she took good care of everyone else, except herself. I sent her a card to thank her for all her help and attention. I likewise told her that I wanted us to be friends forever, but to be able to do that we *both* had to be around. I asked her to think more about herself and take better care of her health, *I* was a prime example that her health needed to be a priority. She was very touched when she received my card and promised to do just that. I am proud and happy to report that she joined Weight Watchers and as of this writing has lost thirty-six pounds. Her doctor is particularly pleased with the reduction in her blood pressure and blood sugar levels, as well as her weight loss. She seems happier and more self confident now since she has lost weight.

CHAPTER 24

Tuesday, August 30, 2011

My follow-up appointment with the cardiologist, Dr. Anil, is scheduled for today. My daughter's appointment is this morning as well. When I went to get dressed, I realized there was another new thing that I had to take into consideration; I had to select clothing that I could wear over my device. The sensors and defibrillator pads added extra bulk around my midriff and back, so I needed to wear clothing that was a bit loose. There was also the wire that went from the garment to the monitor so I could only wear clothes that were in two pieces. My friends joked with me saying that the cable that went from the garment to the monitor looked like I had a tail coming out from under my blouse.

I asked my sister to come with us to the appointment. Dr. Anil checked me over first. One of the first things he told me was if my heart issues had been discovered *before* I had the heart attack, they would have most likely done open-heart surgery.

"If that's the case, then I'm glad that I had the heart attack first," I replied. He said that my heart attack had been a mild one, and I was surprised by that statement. I assumed that it was more severe than mild.

My sister voiced what we were both thinking. "If it was a mild heart attack, why then does she have so much damage?" She asked.

We had deduced that there had been a considerable time lapse between the actual heart attack and my going to the hospital to receive treatment and the doctor used this example to explain it to us.

"It is like when you have a plant that is wilted because it needs watering. If it hasn't been very long since it was watered, and you water it again, it will respond quickly and perk back up. However, the longer that it goes without water the harder it will be for it to come back and that is what has happened with your heart. Since you were not aware that you had a heart attack and you did not seek treatment right away, your heart was without proper blood flow for a considerable time. That is why you have the damage that you have." (Finally, that made perfect sense to me.)

That was where the low ejection fraction came in. The left ventricle (LV) was not contracting properly, its function was now compromised due to lack of proper blood flow for a significant time after the heart attack and without proper treatment. Now my LV was just working at a fraction of what it should and wasn't functioning efficiently. That was why I had been told that I would need reevaluation in three months, possibly for an implantable defibrillator (ICD), in case there was no improvement. I was finally getting the big picture. This was also the reason that my pain was gone when I awoke that Monday morning. The heart attack had left my heart weak and flaccid since the LV was inadequately contracting at that point.

Next, he stressed the importance of my taking the cholesterol medication and I *promised* that I was going to do that faithfully. He told me something else about the cholesterol medication that I didn't know. He said that cholesterol medication served another purpose other than just lowering my cholesterol, as an added benefit it makes the areas in your arteries where there is plaque buildup, smoother. He showed me on a chart how plaque looks when it has ruptured. *Not a pretty sight*! He referred to this as unstable plaque. However, he said by continuing to take the cholesterol medications, unstable plaque can be converted into stable plaque. With stable plaque, it's smoother and less likely to form a clot.

We next discussed my blood pressure, which was *very low*. He wanted it to be low, because it would put less stress on my heart, but he did temporarily cut back on my blood pressure medication. He told me to increase the dosage back to where it had been prescribed originally, *as* I was able to tolerate it. He stressed that the numbers were not as important as the way I felt. He told me as long as I felt good and wasn't dizzy or fainting, not to be overly concerned with the numbers. He wanted me to come back in two months. When I would return, I would have blood work, and an echocardiogram. I scheduled my next appointment for Wednesday, October 26, it would be a *long, long* two months.

Next, it was my daughters turn and we briefly explained what had taken place when she was at the water park. She was also experiencing some chest pain. I guess partly because of what had just happened to me, he decided it best to run several tests. This I felt was probably to put my mind at ease, as well. He had her run a treadmill stress test and ordered an echocardiogram. All tests came back as normal but just to be on the safe side and cover all bases, he sent her home with a Holter monitor. This unit monitors your heart rhythms during daily activity and at rest. It's worn twenty-four hours, and then returned so that the rhythms recorded can be processed and evaluated. We were to return the next day for the results. Mom and daughter now had matching heart monitors. *How cute*!

The next day we were getting ready to go back for my daughter's appointment when, as I was getting dressed, my device started to *siren alarm*. That was the first time the siren alarm had gone off, I pressed the response buttons as instructed, and the treatment was canceled. Of course, it scared me to death (well almost). I had been instructed if that happened, I was to call the 1-800 number. This I did, and after reviewing all my latest data and asking several questions, the technician said that it was from "artifact." I didn't understand what this meant, but I was definitely going to ask the doctor when we went for my daughter's results. The technician on the phone assured me that there *did not* appear to be a problem with my heart. Maybe there wasn't a problem before that alarm went off, but what about *now*, after being scared out of my wits?

I would learn that "artifact" is electrical interference from muscle movement. The electrodes on the device are very sensitive to movement. Since I was getting dressed at the time the alarm went off, that was most likely the cause. When that alarm goes off though, you cannot help but to be absolutely, terrified.

We waited for my daughter's results and it was very good news, everything seemed fine. We still wondered though what would be causing her to have chest pain. The doctor said that since it didn't appear to be her heart, it could be either digestive related or a condition called Costochondritis. This refers to an inflammation of the area where the cartilage at the end of the ribs, joins the breastbone. You have pain with each breath because of the expansion of the rib cage and he decided this was the most probable cause. We were never able to determine why she fainted that day but the bottom line was her heart was healthy, that was all that counted. A few months later, we would learn that her cholesterol was high. She was started on cholesterol medications as a precaution because of *my* history, even though she was only 23.

Thursday, September 8, 2011

My husband was next, I wanted him to have a checkup on his heart too and today he was seeing the doctor who had performed my procedures, Dr. Nair. He had just come back from his trip to India. I thanked him and told him how grateful I was to him for giving me a second chance at the rest of my life. There were a few tense moments due to issues involving my husband's blood pressure. I practically held my breath waiting in anticipation, praying that he didn't have a problem as well. After the doctor performed several tests, he got a good report on his visit. That was great news! I guess it was just me and I was relieved because we didn't need heart problems for anyone else in the family.

It was interesting that around this same time quite a few friends and others who heard about what had happened with me, also scheduled check-ups with a cardiologist. I guess what I had been through, had for good reason, alarmed them and they wanted to prevent being caught off guard as I had been. I joked that I should get a commission for recruiting new business for the cardiologists.

Near this same time as well, I began to hear of a number of heart cases involving people who were *fifty-five years old*. It was very strange (maybe, I just took notice of it more now). My sister and I were discussing this and she had an amusing insight on the matter.

She said, "You know how they say that fifty is the new forty. Well I think perhaps *fifty-five is the new seventy*."

I thought she might possibly be right, at least it sure felt that way. Age fifty-five, it would seem, can be a health turning point for some.

CHAPTER 25

I could hardly wait for my next visit, maybe then I would have some concrete answers, but in the meantime, I tried to keep my mind occupied. I started doing research about my condition on the computer and in books. You've probably figured out by now that I have an inquiring mind, and as they say, "inquiring minds want to know." I've always felt it best to be able to understand what you are dealing with and I *still* feel that it's a good thing. It's important to understand your condition so you can ask intelligent, informed questions. However, this particular circumstance was different. I was in bad physical condition and my emotions were all over the place, as well. The more I read, the more afraid I became. One of the problems was that I didn't fully understand all that I was reading because I wasn't familiar with many of the technical terms used. I would then have to look up the meanings of these terms and then try to figure out the gist of what I was reading. I was trying to interpret things that it takes doctors many years to learn, *without* the benefit of a real instructor. I guess it was sort of like a self-taught course of "Cardiology for Dummies." Much of what I read made me think that my future was a very bleak one, and it frightened me.

Another thing that I didn't even think to take into consideration was one of the books I was using for reference was printed in 1982. It was nearly thirty-year-old information! Tremendous strides have since been made in the field of cardiac medicine. At the time that this book was written, stents were still in the clinical trial stages, not in general use. *A lot* had changed, so much of the information that I was basing my fears on was not even up to date. That is an excellent example of why doing this *can* be dangerous. At last, I recognized this was a mistake at this specific time. I was way too fragile both physically and emotionally for this. My common sense finally kicked in and I came to the realization that I *had* to stop doing research *for now* for my own sanity and health, and I did so. I would advise anyone in the same circumstance to do the same.

Most likely because of the above-mentioned issues, I was having a difficult time sleeping. As I said previously, my bed became my enemy. For one thing, I started having bad dreams, which continued for a while. I think now that they were a side effect of some of my new medications. They eventually went away, I presume, as I got accustomed to the medications. I *didn't* want to go to bed at night because I had a morbid fear of not waking up. I think this mostly stemmed from the fact that I had experienced the heart attack while sleeping. I would try to stay up as long as I possibly could, hoping that being extremely tired, I might fall asleep soon after getting into bed. That way it would give me less time to be stressed-out and pensively think, or should I say, "*over-think*" things.

It was a very difficult time for me because I feared that the worst might not be over even though I sincerely hoped that it was. I would notice myself during daily activities, just sighing for no reason and my moods varied. I also noticed that I had an empty feeling in my chest. It was the same feeling you get when you hear some sort of bad news and was what I would refer to as a "heart sinking feeling." To this very day, I'm not sure if that "feeling" was physical *or* emotional.

Some days I was okay, but some days I felt very depressed. The feelings of sadness and feeling depressed lead to another negative emotion, I felt *guilty* for feeling sad. I had just experienced a life-altering ordeal that could have easily cost me my life. I was aware that I was extremely fortunate and grateful to be alive and I *wanted* to feel happy. I felt that I *should* feel happy not sad and when I didn't it made me feel guilty. I've come to discern that all these feeling were normal under the circumstances, albeit unpleasant. Depression is common after a heart attack or any procedure involving the heart. In fact, it may be up to three times higher than in the general population. Reporting these feelings to our doctors can permit them to support us through these dark, difficult times, perhaps prescribing the appropriate medications to assist in our recovery. Thankfully, that empty feeling and depression eventually did go away.

My husband was still concerned about me being home alone. He worried about me needing help with no one around and decided to have a security system installed that had an ambulance/help button. I hated to admit it out loud, but it did make me feel better knowing that help would be just a push of a button away. When the technician went to install the control panel, my husband asked me where I wanted it mounted. I told him it didn't matter, just to use his own judgment, but I could tell he was not quite satisfied with that answer. After the technician left, he told me it concerned him that I didn't have an opinion about where to install the control panel.

He said, "That's not like you," and it wasn't. I normally had an opinion on everything. He was worried that I'd lost my spirit and was giving up. I told him not to worry, I wasn't giving up. It was just that now I realized that some things aren't so important that I needed to make a big deal over them, as I was seeing things from a different perspective now. I never did need to call for help, but it was reassuring to know that it was there, just in case.

As time passed, one big problem arose was with a claim filed on my health insurance. They were paying only a very small portion on my device rental, due to a small technicality. I had to make many phone calls and write numerous letters in order for them to reverse their decision and pay the claim, a very large claim, I might add. A very kind, helpful woman who worked at the cardiologist's office helped me immensely with this matter. She transcribed a letter from my doctor in order to help to get them to pay. I remember the day she called to let me know the letter was ready.

She said, "I want to warn you, the letter contains some strong wording and we don't want it to scare you, we just want the insurance company to realize how serious this is."

The strong wording that she spoke about were three references that said, *"At high risk for sudden cardiac death."* It was *difficult* and *unsettling* to see in print, but it must have accomplished its intended purpose. I was very grateful that she went the extra mile for me. This whole matter was tremendously stressful to deal with and I was *extremely* upset with the insurance company on several occasions. This I knew was not good for me. Having to deal with a matter like this is something that a person with a weakened heart should not be subjected.

There was one silly instance that I feel compelled to mention. Despite *all* that had taken place, it seemed I had to develop a new mind-set. For one fleeting moment, it escaped me that from here on out, I was now and *forever* considered a heart patient. I know that sounds crazy, how could I overlook that?

One afternoon in a conversation with my husband as I referred to my nitroglycerin pills, I said as soon as I got *better*, I was going to give them to one of our friends, another heart patient. As soon as the words left my mouth, it hit me like a ton of bricks. Even while I might improve, I will *always* have heart disease, and I may *always* need them. I *didn't* like that new realization, but I would have to accept it.

CHAPTER 26

You may be wondering as time passed how things were working out with my device. Allow me to provide an update on that subject. There were several episodes where the siren alarm sounded and when this did happen, I felt completely unnerved. When you hear that audible warning that a treatment is about to be delivered, there simply are no words to describe *exactly* how you feel inside. Well, perhaps the words, *"absolute, unbridled terror"* would be semi-appropriate. I would press the response buttons as instructed, and hope beyond hope that it worked. I can't imagine anyone in that position *not* being afraid. The ironic thing was, I was even afraid to be afraid, fearful that the extreme fear I was feeling would cause an arrhythmia, and that made me more afraid. It was such a crazy, vicious cycle.

We finally found the underlying cause of several of the alarm warnings. The woman, who had instructed me on the use of the device, had told me it was common for a person's skin to get irritated where the sensors rubbed. She told me if this should happen, to apply a little petroleum jelly under the sensors. After a short time, I did experience some skin irritation and decided to try the petroleum jelly. I would apply it after my bath, just before putting the device back on, I noticed that the alarms seem to occur shortly after this. Of course, this always happened at night, right before bedtime, something I *really* didn't need at that specific time to unnerve me. Once this would take place, I just couldn't get to sleep due to the rush of adrenalin. With the assistance of one of the representatives on the help line, we were able to figure out what was causing the problem. I was incorrectly informed; petroleum jelly was *not* to be used. It caused the sensors to slide excessively, giving the monitor the impression of an abnormal rhythm. When I finally discovered this, I decided I would prefer raw skin to being scared out of my wits. *That* solved that problem.

My device seemed to be a novelty everywhere I went since it appeared that no one had heard of it before. Everyone had many questions about it and I was now the "popular girl with the cool, new toy." I would notice strangers taking notice of it, given that they couldn't help but see the red blinking light on the front. It was obvious most people were very curious and I would usually explain to satisfy their curiosity. There was even one friend that I played a practical joke on. He would always ask me about my device every time I saw him; I would then grab him by the arm, shaking it while making a buzzing sound. I got a funny reaction from him, but I promise he was the only person I played that joke on.

There was only one person I met in a restaurant, who had an inkling as to what it was. She noticed it and questioned me about it. After talking with her, I found out that she had serious heart issues and was awaiting a heart transplant. Sadly, a year later I read in the obituaries that she had lost her fight.

Then, there were some people who were literally afraid to be around me and my next-door neighbor was one of them. She is frightened of *anything* medical. She hates to go to the doctor, and says that she *jumps* when the doctor gets close to her with a stethoscope. It made her nervous to even be near me. I explained that she could not get shocked unless it was delivering a treatment and she was touching me; nevertheless, she made it a point to stay as far away as she could.

However, one day I had walked outside as she was leaving for work. We were just chatting when a siren alarm went off. I started walking back towards my house because I needed to be close to the charger unit, which also transmitted data. I told her not to leave me because I was trying to figure out the cause of the alarm this time.

She followed me, looking completely frightened and in a small, fearful voice asked, "What do you want me to do?"

"I'm trying to figure out what the problem is, just stay with me until I know if everything is okay, or if you need to call 911," I said.

I honestly think if she had actually needed to call 911, we would have probably needed *two* ambulances, one for me and one for her. She was so funny and to this day insists that wearing the device was harder on her, than it was on me. I would beg to differ on that point.

In time, we would figure out the problem that day was most likely caused by electromagnetic interference. At the same time that I was outside, there was a garbage truck near my house and the alarm went off just as it started to grind up the garbage. Something similar did happen on two other occasions. After doing some research, we concluded that electromagnetic interference was the most logical answer we could find. The manual stated that many common devices including motors, as well as electronic equipment might produce electromagnetic interference that can affect its operation. Now can you understand why I worried so much about it *malfunctioning*?

It was something that *really* took a lot of getting used to. Another thing to get used to was every time I went somewhere, I had to unplug and take my charger unit with me. This fit in a large tote bag that I carried everywhere I went. I needed the charger just in case I had an alarm since my charger was necessary in order to transmit the data. That was the only way I could be sure if it was a *real alarm* or a *false alarm*. This was one gigantic hassle.

I *was* allowed to drive while wearing the device; though, I did not like doing so. I just drove a few times while wearing it, and only for short distances. The reason I didn't want to drive while wearing it was because I felt like I would be a hazard on the road. Every time it alarmed, it upset me so much that I was afraid if it would alarm while I was driving I would cause an accident.

This may surprise you but there was one thing that changed over time. I somewhere along the way went from calling it my *"bomb"* to calling it my *"box."* I guess that made it seem less threatening; after all, it was ultimately for my protection. It was in actuality my *guardian*. I was even getting used to sleeping with it, given that I eventually learned how to position it in order for sleeping to be more comfortable. At the beginning, I wondered *how* I was *ever* going to wear it the entire time, but as my appointment for the echocardiogram neared; I realized I was going to make it.

This device was technology at its *finest*. When I think how far technology has progressed, I am so impressed. I couldn't help but think about people in the past, as I realized the fact that numerous people could have benefitted from a device like this. Before this device was widely available, countless went home unprotected and I imagine some died and that thought makes me feel sad. I do feel fortunate and grateful that I had it accessible for my use. As difficult as it was to wear, I'm thankful that my doctor was truly concerned enough to prescribe it for me.

As time has passed, I've learned that silly memories can come from serious events. You sometimes need silly things to break the tension, accordingly never underestimate the powerful healing effect of humor. My mother and I started a new routine during this time that we continue even now.

Several years ago, there was a classic commercial for a hospital on television. It featured a married couple, who over the course of several commercials would take turns hiding from each other. When the unsuspecting party would walk by, the other would jump out of hiding, yell, and scare their mate. You would see that they looked very frightened and they would then stop and grab their chest over their heart. As they stood there, breathing hard, the other person (who had jumped out) would say, "You good?" They would nod and say "yes." The ending punch line was, "There's a better way to have your heart checked." The spokesperson then instructed the audience to make an appointment with the hospital/sponsor. As I said, it was a classic and very funny. Many people remember it as one of their favorites. It was because of that commercial that now every time my mother or I call each other, when the other answers we say, "*You good?*" It always brings a smile to our faces ... and that does our hearts "good."

CHAPTER 27

I was feeling better by this time, both physically as well as emotionally; I felt deep inside that I was stronger. I knew the results of the echocardiogram were going to be the determining factor. It was going to say "yea" or "nay" as to the direction my life would be taking. Even though I felt that I was stronger, I didn't want to get my hopes up. I certainly didn't want to be disappointed. After all, I hadn't been a good judge of my own health in the recent past; I had a heart attack and didn't even realize it. I guess the best description for the way that I felt would be, *hopefully optimistic*.

My only complaint at this point was some tightness in my chest that would come and go. It wasn't horrible but it was at times uncomfortable, and a bit disquieting. I hadn't acquired my full strength back yet either because I still limited my exertion since I really didn't know exactly what was going on inside me. I was fairly active around the house, but still didn't do any heavy lifting.

I continued to dislike the idea of having an implanted defibrillator. As with most new and unpleasant ideas, you do become more used to and/or accepting of them as time passes. I gave it much thought and decided if the tests showed that it was absolutely necessary, then that was what I would have to do. I had come too far to refuse it, if it was in fact, what I really needed.

There was one other aspect to consider. What if there had been only a *small* improvement? What was I to do then? At this point, my health insurance company was now paying at 100%. My appointment was for October 26. I had only two months before we would have to start *all over* again with the deductible and out of pocket minimums. If the improvement was only a small one, should I go ahead and have the procedure done while the insurance company was paying the lion's share of the medical expenses? I did have to consider our finances. The other option was to give my heart more time to recover, perhaps then, I wouldn't need a defibrillator. I *had* to be practical, but I didn't want to have a medical procedure that was unnecessary. I was just going to have to wait for my results in order to make that final decision.

I remember feeling very on edge and nervous the day before my echocardiogram. This day seemed to be the longest yet in view of the fact that the unknown can drive you crazy. After the extended wait, I just *needed* answers.

***

Wednesday, October 26, 2011

The red-letter day that I had been *waiting* for had *finally* arrived and again, I was wondering what my future held. I had two appointments that day; the first was early in the morning for blood work to check my cholesterol levels and liver enzymes. They were also going to perform the *long anticipated* echocardiogram, as well. My next appointment was after lunch to get all my test results. After my morning appointment, I was so anxious to get back to learn my fate. It seemed so long that I had waited in expectation for this day. I can remember at first even wishing to be able to stay asleep for these months until this day would arrive, in just a few more hours, I would have some of the answers that I had long awaited. I went back home and took a nap while waiting, thinking that would make time *seem* to go by faster.

My husband came home in order to accompany me to my afternoon appointment. I was glad that he was with me, just in case the news was *not* the news that I wanted to hear. As we waited in the waiting room, I noticed a woman wearing scrubs. Her scrubs bore a logo, which I recognized as being from the company that manufactured my device, so I approached her and we got into a conversation. She was there to see my doctor and had my compliance report with her. It showed that I had worn the device 98% of the time, the other 2% was bath time. The doctor would know from this, that I had worn it as instructed.

When my doctor came in, he was all smiles. I took that as a good sign and he didn't make me wait long to hear the good news. He said that my ejection fraction, which was less than 20%, when I left the hospital, was now 55%. A normal ejection fraction was within the range of 50%-60%. The echocardiogram showed that everything had improved and looked good. To say that we were *thrilled* was an *understatement* since there simply are not enough adjectives to describe how I felt. I think this *must* be what it feels like to win the lottery; I couldn't have received better news! He also said I could stop wearing my device and send it back; this was double the good news in one day. I told the doctor that my wedding anniversary was in two days and this good news was *all* I wanted for an anniversary present this year. This was the best present ever!

Once again, he told me if my problems had been discovered before my heart attack, I would have most likely had open-heart surgery. It is interesting to see how things can work out for us in the end, even if we don't realize it at the time. By the time that my angiogram was performed, my heart was in such a weakened state, open-heart surgery would have been a greater risk. That's why stents were the better option and I wasn't going to argue with that.

I knew now that I could completely forgive myself for not recognizing my symptoms in advance. This was truly a blessing in disguise since things really had worked out for the best in the end. I fully realized that I had dodged a bullet. My heart was able to recover from the damage caused by the heart attack. Of course, never having a heart attack in the first place would have been preferable.

We next discussed my blood work. My total cholesterol was within normal range, but my HDL (good cholesterol) was low, he wanted to try to increase this.

He wrote me a new prescription for my cholesterol medication, changing it from 40 milligrams to 80 milligrams. I didn't really want him to increase it that much, that quickly, out of concern over possible side effects. However, I didn't question him about it; I was on such a natural high because of the good news that I had just received.

I told him I felt good; my only complaint was tightness in my chest that would come and go. He said that this might go away in time. He wanted me to increase my activity level and told me to do whatever I felt like I could do, and not to let *anyone* tell me otherwise.

We were ecstatic! We left the office once again hand in hand, again thinking that we were good. We hoped it would not be dé jà vu—*all over again*. We wanted to celebrate so we indulged in a guilty pleasure. We went for beignets and coffee. They were good, but not as good as it was going to feel to go home and finally take off this "box," forevermore.

Of course, you may have noticed that I have this little habit of over thinking everything. There was this nagging thought in the back of my mind that I couldn't help but think. "What if I still might need my device? It had only been two and a half months since the heart attack." I was remarkably surprised that I was thinking that way. I truly *hated* this contrivance at first, but as time passed, had come to accept it as a part of my recovery process. It had been my guardian for all this time. I knew that I wouldn't miss *it* per se, but I would miss the *security* it provided, in that it was a protection for me. It did seem strange without it that first night; however, I quickly adjusted to its absence. I didn't grieve for it for very long. I sent the device back the very next day. My only regret is that I didn't take a picture while wearing it, just for a keepsake. It is exceedingly strange how our feelings can change with time.

CHAPTER 28

As I thought about my doctor increasing my cholesterol medication, I did have apprehension. I was concerned that doubling it would be too much of a jump and I didn't want any additional problems. I considered just taking one and a half of my former strength, 60 milligrams instead of 80 milligrams. After a great deal of contemplation, I then reasoned on the matter. "What if when I come back my numbers still aren't right? Then I'll have to tell the doctor I didn't follow his instructions. Not listening to my doctor's advice is what got me into this trouble in the first place." For that reason, I decided to take the medication *exactly* as he had instructed me to. As I have stated before, I *do not* like repeating my mistakes.

Friday, October 28, 2011

Today was our special day, our thirty-ninth wedding anniversary. We celebrated in a simple way by going out to dinner together. That night we reflected on all the things that had transpired in the last three months. It had been a crazy roller coaster ride, but we were still here ... together ... and still sane for the *most part*. We were happy and grateful that everything had turned out as well as it had. We both had a renewed appreciation for the gift of life and each other. It was indeed a special anniversary, just knowing all we had been through as a couple to get to this point, made it even more precious to us.

For the next three weeks, I felt really good. I was starting to feel like my old self again, which was wonderful! Then I noticed I had a back and neck ache and the discomfort was significant. I likewise observed that the tightness in my chest was happening more frequently and was getting stronger. In addition, at times I had shortness of breath as well. I *didn't* like what I was feeling; it brought back bad memories of the time right before my heart attack. It wasn't as severe as it had been then, but it was very disturbing to me. I felt these symptoms for about a week. However, I knew that it hadn't even been a month since all my tests showed that my heart was *supposed* to be fine. I really didn't know what was happening. Was I just over reacting? I wasn't sure what to believe.

Tuesday, November 22, 2011

My annual gynecology appointment was scheduled that day with the nurse practitioner. She was unaware of anything that had happened to me over the last few months and when she asked how I had been doing, I had much to tell her. She wanted to know how I was feeling now. I told her I had been feeling good up until about a week ago. I said the pain in my neck and shoulders reminded me of the way I felt before the heart attack, but I was supposed to be fine. She told me if she were in my place, she would go back to have it checked out.

"From what you told me," she began, "you didn't have typical symptoms last time, that being the case, I would definitely have these pains checked out."

I did tell her there was one positive thing about my heart attack. I no longer had any hot flashes; my heart attack had fixed that problem. I'm not really sure why, and she wasn't either, except she thought it may have something to do with my weight loss. I feel it may be related to some of the medications that I am now taking. But, who knows?

I left her office wondering whether I should go home or go to the cardiologist's office. I sat in my car for a little while contemplating what would be the best thing to do. I really didn't want to go, but last time I'd made a few wrong decisions and didn't want a repeat of that. I needed to make the right decision *this* time. I decided it might be best to go straight to the cardiologist's office to inquire if Dr. Anil could see me. Once in his office I discovered that he was at the hospital performing a procedure at the time. The cardiologist that had put my stents in, Dr. Nair was also unavailable that day. The receptionist told me that she could work me in with another cardiologist. I had never seen this doctor before, but I was willing to wait.

I was able to see the new doctor and after talking with him, he decided to have me run a stress test on the treadmill. That was the *most* that I had exerted myself in a long time, I had never even tried to run since the heart attack. I was able to stay on the treadmill for only seven and a half minutes. I went back in to meet with the doctor. He told me they weren't able to get my heart rate up to where they wanted it to be, so I would need additional tests. He wanted me to come back the next day for a nuclear stress test, also called nuclear perfusion. This test combines nuclear scanning along with exercise in order to check blood flow to the heart muscle, and assess heart function. They were in effect, checking to be certain there were no new blockages in my stents, put in three months earlier. The nurse instructed me *not* to take my usual dose of the beta-blocker medication that night or the one for the next morning. A beta-blocker slows the heart rate and decreases the strength of each heartbeat. Some of the reasons they prescribe these medications are because it lowers your blood pressure and reduces the stress on the heart. They wanted to see what my heart would do under stress without these medications in my system. I was given other specific instructions to follow for the test.

I then scheduled my appointment for the nuclear stress test. It was going to be administered tomorrow afternoon, Wednesday, November 23. I was to receive the results of this test at my following appointment, scheduled for Friday, November 25.

"What if they should discover something serious, will someone tell me that day or do I still have to wait until Friday?" I inquired.

"Don't worry, if something serious is detected you won't be allowed to leave," she told me.

I *presumed* that was a good thing.

CHAPTER 29

Wednesday, November 23, 2011

I arrived for my scheduled appointment for the nuclear stress test and my younger daughter had come with me. The office was nearly empty today, with just a fraction of the usual staff working because tomorrow would be Thanksgiving holiday. I didn't have a long wait before the technician called me to the back.

The nuclear stress test or nuclear perfusion is performed in three parts. First, in order to allow the radioactive tracer material to be injected, an IV was started in my arm. This would stay in place until the test was completed. Next, while it's at rest, pictures of my heart were taken. As the radioactive material travels via the bloodstream, into the coronary arteries and then the heart muscle, the scanner detects the radiation released and produces a computer image of the heart. Since blood doesn't show up on the scanner, the nuclear material acts as a tracer in the blood. You have to remain very still for about fifteen minutes on a narrow table as the CT scanner scans the chest area.

For the second part of the test, EKG electrodes were attached to my chest. This was so that my blood pressure and heart could be monitored during this phase of the test. Before starting, the technician advised me that the speed and incline would be increased every three minutes. I was told that it was important to stay on the treadmill for as long as I could and when my heart rate reached a certain point, radioactive material would again, be injected through the IV. Once this was injected, I was to try to continue walking for as long as I possibly could, this would yield the most accurate results. My blood pressure and heart rate readings were to be taken for five minutes after I got off the treadmill. The treadmill started, and I did okay for the first three minutes, but it did seem somewhat harder than the day before. Then, as the speed and incline was raised, I found it getting *considerably* more difficult. I had been able to walk for seven and a half minutes the day before; this was feeling significantly more intense today. In reality, I was having doubts as to whether I would be able to stay on for that long today. The technicians were helping by cheering me on. At five and a half minutes, I warned them that I couldn't go much longer. At six minutes, I was injected for the second time with the radioactive material. They encouraged me to *try* to continue walking for as long as I could. I walked for another thirty seconds and felt very weak. I told them that I needed to get off, ***NOW!***

She stopped the treadmill and sat me in a waiting chair. Normally the treadmill is slowed down gradually in order for you to recover and cool down. I had to get off immediately, or they were going to have to pick me up off the floor. I could just imagine myself fainting, and being flung off the back of the treadmill.

I felt awful; my chest was extremely tight and felt like it was going to implode. I was breathing shallowly and in tremendous pain.

They asked if I was okay and I replied that I wasn't. I told them I was having severe chest and back pain. One of the technicians offered to give me nitroglycerin spray for the chest pains, but the other technician warned her not to because my blood pressure was 90/50. I didn't know exactly why it was so low, but *I* thought after running for six and a half minutes, my blood pressure should have been higher than that. Nitroglycerin will further lower the blood pressure; I didn't need that at this moment.

I was in pain and felt exceedingly fearful. I thought that the stress test might have brought on another heart attack due to the intense pain I was feeling. Years ago, my mother had a cousin who had a heart attack while having a stress test, and he died right there in the doctor's office. I asked the technician if the chair leaned back because I was extremely uncomfortable. It did, and after resting a while, I *gradually* began to feel somewhat better. I wanted to know if the short interval that I walked after the last injection, had been enough time to obtain the results they needed. They told me yes, but I'm still not really sure about that one.

As I said earlier, this was the day before a big holiday and there was just a small staff working today. Nine cardiologists regularly work out of this office, but there was only one cardiologist in-house today. He had been notified about the difficulties that took place during the nuclear perfusion.

It was now time for the concluding part of the test. Once more, I had to stay very still while pictures were taken of my heart, this time under stress conditions. This again took about fifteen minutes and the entire time I was deeply concerned. I knew that it hadn't gone well even though I didn't know *exactly* what it all meant. I wondered what was going to happen now. I was supposed to be all right; at least I was less than a month ago. After the pictures were completed, I went back to the waiting area with my daughter.

Not long after I returned to the waiting area, my mother arrived. She wanted to come with me earlier, but had another appointment to keep that afternoon. As soon as her appointment was over, she came to meet us. I told her that I didn't think it had gone well and filled her in on what had taken place. Shortly, we were directed to a small room in the back of the office. We met with a nurse who told us that the in-house doctor had reviewed the test findings and wanted me to go *directly* to the hospital for an angiogram. I sighed deeply and felt profoundly distressed, again. *I definitely didn't want this.* Nevertheless, what choice did I have? I wondered what had gone wrong in such a short time. Could it be another blockage so soon? I thought I was on the mend. I thought that I was moving in the right direction, but was I? I simply had no idea at this point. While the staff got my paperwork ready, I tearfully called my husband to let him know what was happening and he assured me he would be right there.

CHAPTER 30

My mother drove me to the hospital, which was about two blocks away. As instructed, we went in through the emergency room. I was seated in a wheel chair and wheeled towards the cath lab. Again, so many unpleasant thoughts were going through my mind. I started to cry; I was very afraid again. I didn't know what to expect as to the outcome. I thought that all this bad stuff was behind me. I had no time to prepare or adjust to this new unwelcomed development.

At the far end of the hall, I could see a man in royal blue scrubs walking towards us and as he got closer, I recognized that it was my old friend, George. The cath lab had just received my paper work from the doctor's office.

"I thought that your name sounded familiar." He saw that I was crying and lightheartedly said, "What is this? We don't allow crying here in the cath lab. This has got to stop."

I admitted that I felt better already knowing that *he* was there. My mother told him that we were going to have to get a cardboard cutout of him for me to keep at home, for when I didn't feel good. (*Seriously, he probably could sell tons of these.*) He just laughed. I then asked which cardiologist was going to perform the angiogram today. It was Dr. Nair; the same doctor who had performed my two previous procedures. I felt better knowing that too. I knew that he was a very capable doctor and already familiar with my past issues.

Next, I was brought to a holding area to be prepped, and an IV was started. The nurses asked several questions about my medications, they wanted to be certain that I had been taking the blood thinners, as instructed. *Then*, out came the consent forms and they started to explain them to me again. I told them I knew exactly what they had to say. *Here I was doing this all over again*! I asked if it were possible for blockages to happen so soon; it had only been three and a half months. They said, it was possible and had happened before. I learned that it was not uncommon for people to have problems of this nature early on. I erroneously thought because I was taking the medications as instructed and watching my diet that other blockages wouldn't be a concern, until perhaps *years* down the road.

By this time, my husband had arrived. Perhaps my family was putting on a brave face for me, but everyone seemed to be in good spirits. I said my "I love you's" and I was off to the cath lab, *again*. Everything was happening *so fast* and I didn't have time to fully mentally process, all that was taking place. I was understandably nervous and upset by these recent events.

When he pushed the gurney into the cath lab suite, George said, "Does this look familiar?"

Unfortunately it did. Again, all were going about their jobs in the calm, laid-back manner as before. Apparently, I was the only one who was stressed-out and I guess if it had to be any of us, then *I* was the best candidate.

Once more, I was back on the narrow, hard table. My left arm was being stretched out and strapped down as they were planning to go through my left radial artery. I was yet again, being draped with the sterile drapes and some type of plastic. The anesthetist who was in the process of numbing my wrist noticed my incision scar from my first angiogram.

"I can see that you've been here before," he commented.

"Yes I'm a frequent flyer it seems, three times in three months," I confessed.

Someone spoke up and said, "That's nothing, there've been some people who have been back here thirty times."

I adamantly replied, "Well I don't want to be one of *those* people!"

I again asked that they take good care of me, which essentially translates into, "Please see to it that I wake up." I even decided to sweeten the pot. I told them if they took extra good care of me, I would bake them all brownies. That idea seemed like a big hit; as it never hurts to use the currency that works.

Next, the doctor came in, walked around the table and tried to put me at ease. I *personally* felt that they weren't expecting the outcome to be very positive. They didn't tell me this; it was just a feeling that I had. Here I was once more, not knowing what my future held. As you are well aware, I had such a dread of open-heart surgery. Would my fear be realized this time? This time my conscious sedation was *not* conscious at all.

It was *total* lights out… Again…!

The next thing I remember, I was in a regular room and my family was there with me. My family later told me that I was talking when I came out of the cath lab. They even rode up in the elevator with me to my room, all the while I carried on a big conversation. I don't remember *any* of that! I remember someone bringing me my dinner and *nothing* before. During this brief *lapse of memory*, I even volunteered my daughter, the one who works at the hospital, to bake a cake for one of her co-workers. *See what can happen when you take drugs!*

I was anxious to know what they had discovered during the angiogram. My family told me that everything seemed fine, the stents were all good and there were no new blockages. Everything looked just as it did during my last angiogram. That was welcome news. There were still the blockages in the distal portions of the coronary arteries (the blockages at the bottom of my heart, where the arteries narrow). The doctor felt that *perhaps* these blockages were the cause of my chest tightness and back pain. He added two new medicines to my already long list of medications. One was to relax and widen the blood vessels so that blood could flow more easily to the heart. The other was to improve how well the heart uses oxygen so that it can do more work with less oxygen.

The doctor also wanted me to stop taking my cholesterol medication and start a different one. It was my family who had spoken with the doctor after the angiogram, so I wanted to know why he was making this change, but they were uncertain. When the nurse came around to discharge me, I asked her the same question, but she didn't know either. I was very, very happy that there were no new blockages found. I was so pleased that no further surgery or procedures were necessary. However, something just didn't add up to me. The blockages in the distal areas had *always* been there. Why were they starting to cause me pain ... *now*?

CHAPTER 31

I remembered telling Dr. Anil a month earlier that I had *a little tightness* in my chest, but this *specific combination* of discomfort had started about three weeks *after* I had seen him. I felt like, if it *had* been caused by the distal blockages, that I would have had it from the start. I thought about him changing my cholesterol medication on my last visit and I wondered if perhaps it *may* have something to do with my issues. It was changed from 40 milligrams to 80 milligrams only a month earlier.

After being discharged from the hospital, I had the new medications filled that Dr. Nair had prescribed and started taking them that night, with the exception of the new cholesterol medicine. I also stopped the former cholesterol medication, as instructed and decided *not* to start the new one right away. I figured I'd stay off of it for a few days in order give my body a break. The next day, I called the pharmacy to inquire about how long it would take to get that medication out of my system. They said it would take about two to three weeks; I just had a *nagging* feeling about the cholesterol medication. The following day there was *no* change in the chest pain or shortness of breath. I had hoped that the new medications would bring *quick relief* and improvement, but they did not.

A week later, I fulfilled my promise to the guys in the cath lab by baking them a huge pan of brownies. If I was going to be a *regular*, I wanted to stay on their good side. The next day, which was eight days after the angiogram, I went *back* to see the cardiologist because I was still having *all* the same symptoms. I wanted to know how long before I could expect to see an improvement. I felt like the new medications should be working by now. I likewise wanted to know if there was *anything else* that I should know about the angiogram findings since I hadn't talked with the cardiologist myself.

I didn't discover anything *new*, just what I had learned at the hospital. I wondered as well, why I had experienced such difficulties during the nuclear perfusion test; the data gathered during the test had indicated that there were blockages again in the arteries of my heart. That was the reason I was sent straight to the hospital for the angiogram. I would learn this was due to a false-positive result on the test. I don't know precisely the reason that this occurred in my case, but I've learned that it does happen on occasion. Despite the fact that it scared me out of my wits, I was *relieved* that it wasn't an actual new blockage.

The week before when I had gone to the gynecologist, she asked me about residual heart damage and I told her that I wasn't sure. I knew that my ejection fraction had come up, but I didn't know about other remaining damage. I told the cardiologist of our conversation and inquired about an answer. He took his time and sifted through all my records. He looked up with a pleased look on his face and said that there remained "no appreciable damage." I asked him if that was typical, to go from where I was when I left the hospital to where I was now in such a short time. He told me that it was *not* typical and that I had indeed been very fortunate. He assured me that everything was fine, to continue taking the new medications and I agreed to do so.

I continued to have chest pains and shortness of breath for about another two weeks. Then, I began to notice a major improvement in the way I was feeling; I was starting to feeling normal again. It was a welcome feeling, but it only lasted about a week. I would get my hopes up and then the chest, neck and back pain would return, as well as the tightness and shortness of breath. I just wanted to feel good again, to feel normal and not be in pain. I certainly hoped that this was not the "new normal" for me.

I still had nagging doubts about the cholesterol medications causing my pain and started to do research on the computer. From the things I was reading, I concluded that it was very possible that my issues *were* being caused by the medication. I discovered that most people who experienced problems, had muscle pain in their legs. However, chest pain was also a possibility; it just wasn't as common. It was now the end of December and because of all the issues I was experiencing, I decided to stop taking the new cholesterol medication and made *another* appointment with Dr. Anil. That appointment was scheduled for January 4, 2012.

I really hated to be thought of as a chronic complainer. It seemed as if I was becoming a broken record, *always* with the same complaint. I *just* wanted to *feel good* so that I could get on with my life. I was concerned that my doctor would assume that I was a bored housewife who had now become a hypochondriac. I didn't want him to think that I had nothing to do except focus on myself. I knew for a certainty that wasn't the case; I really hoped that he did too.

After all, I didn't go to the doctor unless I felt it was a *necessity*. I think that I *more than proved* that point in the weeks preceding my heart attack. I went in for my appointment on January 4 and told him I thought that the cholesterol medication was not agreeing with me. He said there were many different statin drugs out there, and we were *going* to find the one that would work for me. He said there was a new one on the market and he would give me some samples. His compassion was evident; he was trying his best to help me.

Each time I started a new medication, I really dreaded doing so because I felt apprehensive as to how I would react to it. I felt like I was a human guinea pig, since unfortunately, there was no way to tell how my body was going to respond to it, other than to try taking the medication. I would then just have to wait and see, and hope for the best.

About three weeks after stopping the previous medication, I noticed that I was starting to feel normal again. I took that to mean that it was now was out of my system. When this would happen, I would step up my activity level, and it felt *so good* to be able to do so. I also knew that getting more exercise would also help to lower my cholesterol levels; due to this, I wanted to increase my activity. I began to notice that there seemed to be a pattern forming. I became aware that my issues would start after being on the medications for about three to four weeks. I also observed that it seemed to me, the amount of time that it took for me *start* hurting, it would then take *about* the same amount of time to *stop*. When the pains would start, my activity level would then subsequently drop because I felt especially winded when I tried to exercise.

I recalled the *start* of these problems, they started *before* my last angiogram, and three weeks *after* the doctor increased the dosage of my cholesterol medicine. Had this medication been the cause of me needing another angiogram? Of course, I wasn't sure about that, but the idea of it was disturbing to me. If that *was* the case, it was *very* ironic. Not taking cholesterol medicine had likely caused me to have blockages that resulted in a heart attack and put me in the hospital. Had actually taking the medication caused me to be hospitalized as well? That seemed like a no-win situation to me.

This was unsettling to me since angiography is an invasive procedure with certain risks. I would learn though, that while there *are* risks involved, it is a relatively safe procedure. The risk of serious complications is very low considering the procedure is being performed on patients with heart disease. I would also learn that wrist catheterization is an even safer procedure, provided the cardiologist has sufficient experience with this specific technique. With wrist catheterization, and especially the left wrist, there is less chance of bleeding complications. This is desirable because cardiac patients are usually taking blood thinners. The patient is also able to be mobile sooner, which results in earlier discharge from the hospital and a faster recovery time.

I had been taking my *newest* cholesterol medication for three weeks and I felt fine ... It was then four weeks and everything was still good, I thought *maybe* we had stumbled on the *right* medication this time. Another week passed, it was now week five and that was when it hit and *started* causing me problems. It took longer this time, but it felt like all the other times. I decided that I would *again* stop taking it and just see how things went. I stayed off the medication for three weeks, but was *still* in pain. I felt so discouraged and as much as I hated to, I needed to go *back* to the doctor for his input. This whole scenario was getting so old.

I told my doctor that these pains in my neck and back really concerned and frightened me. It reminded me of the pains that I had for the two weeks prior to my heart attack. I hoped that he understood that I wasn't just being paranoid. I told him I was afraid that I couldn't distinguish between *this* pain and the pain that precedes a heart attack since there was so much similarity between the two. My doctor told me that I shouldn't worry; he said that I would *know*. "What ever told you last time that you should go to the hospital will tell you again," he said. *That* was the problem. This was no comfort to me since I didn't realize last time. It was because of the fact that I *didn't realize*, that I didn't seek medical attention until eighteen to twenty hours later. I certainly didn't want to repeat that mistake and risk heart damage.

He reviewed all my records and asked me a number of questions. His conclusion was that the pain was not heart related, but rather muscular in nature. He felt like I might benefit from taking a muscle relaxer and wanted me to see my family doctor for him to prescribe muscle relaxers for me. He also wanted to know how long I had been off the cholesterol medications, and I told him it had been three weeks. He said if it had been that long and I was still in pain, it probably wasn't the cholesterol medication causing the problem and to resume taking it.

    I *liked* hearing that he felt that my problems were *not* heart related; this was a relief. Nonetheless, I knew something was making me feel this way, I just wished that I knew exactly what that was.

CHAPTER 32

I made an appointment the next day with my family doctor and gave him a brief synopsis of my doctor's visit from the day before. I let him know the cardiologist thought that my issues were muscular in nature and wanted me to resume the cholesterol medications. My family doctor wanted to know how long it had been since I had stopped taking the cholesterol meds, and I told him three weeks. *He* thought that perhaps it was *not* out of my system yet and that *it* may in fact be the culprit causing my problems. He wanted me to stay off it for a few weeks longer. In addition, he gave me a prescription for a mild muscle relaxer.

I now had two completely different opinions, from two different doctors. To whom should I listen? There are times when you just have to go with your gut. Since three weeks had already gone by, I figured I would wait a few more just to see what would happen. I tried taking the muscle relaxers, but I didn't find they gave me any relief. After two more weeks I started to feel good again, the pain was gone *again*. It took a total of five weeks for that to happen. With taking this particular medication, it also took five weeks before I started to feel pain.

Perhaps I was on to something, my theory was that it seemed whatever time it took before the pain started, it would then take the same amount of time for it to go away. I had marked these dates down on the calendar, and I was definitely seeing a pattern here. I went another week without taking the medication just to be sure. I felt great, just like a *normal* person again.

I knew however, because of my past blockages, I *shouldn't* stay off cholesterol medication for an extended time as it had now been six weeks since I stopped taking it. Before starting something new, out of curiosity, I decided it best to have my cholesterol checked. So much had changed since the old days before my heart attack. In the last seven months, I had lost twenty-six pounds due to the fact that I was eating so much better than I used to. I *really was* watching my diet now. I had done some research on natural ways to lower cholesterol and was trying to put that information into practice. When I went in for the cholesterol test, I expected to see a *major improvement* over my past readings.

I was utterly shocked and disappointed when the nurse called with my results. *Even with all these changes*, my total cholesterol was 230. How could it still be that high? Before the heart attack, it was usually between 230 and 240. I felt that *nothing* had changed *despite* all my efforts. I felt so disheartened because I had been working so hard to make improvements. Nonetheless, it did make it apparent just how much I needed the cholesterol medication; this was the concrete proof that I could not deny. I didn't know exactly what to do though. I felt it was causing me physical pain, but I knew I needed to take it. I didn't want to be back where I was before the heart attack. More to the point, I needed to be *even more* careful now that I had stents. This was quite distressing and discouraging, but I refused to let it get the best of me, I had been through too much in the past few months to let that happen. As I've always told my children, "There is *always* another way to do something. There is always *something else* out there that will work." *I just needed to find what that was.*

I had talked with my mother about the cholesterol medication that my father was taking. She told me that the first one he tried *didn't* agree with him, but the next one that his doctor prescribed was the one that worked for him. She said his doctor had told her that my father's medication was one of the older statins, and many people had success with it. I wondered, since I seemed to have inherited his heart problems, perhaps I had inherited his tolerance of this medication as well. I knew it may be a long shot, but I had to do *something*. I called the doctor's office and specifically asked if he would consider prescribing for me the same medication that my father was taking. The nurse said she would speak with him and call me back.

When she did call back, she said that he had agreed to the change, but wanted me to come in for blood work in three weeks. The other thing that pleased me was he was starting me off on a low dose. He had prescribed only 10 milligrams. In some of the research I had done, that was one of the suggestions, to start low and work up in order to build up a tolerance. In addition, I had done some reading about the benefits of CO-Q10. My doctor had approved of this from the beginning, but I had only been taking it sporadically so I decided to take it on the same schedule that I take my prescription medicines. I started taking it *faithfully*, morning and night.

When I went back for my blood work three weeks later, I was surprised again, this time in a good way. With taking only 10 milligrams of the statin, my total cholesterol had gone from 230 down to 183. I was very pleased and the added benefit was that I wasn't hurting yet either. This trend would continue. My next regular scheduled appointment was June 20, 2012, I continued to feel good with no chest or back pain.

When I went for my regular appointment, I had blood work done again. When I saw the results, I was very excited. All my cholesterol numbers were within normal ranges. I thought that I had finally found the answer in this new medicine. On the other hand, my doctor would burst that bubble *somewhat*.

My LDL cholesterol was 122. Normal reference range was less than 130; consequently, I thought that my cholesterol was where it needed to be. My doctor explained that those were *normal ranges* and didn't include values for those at high-risk, which I now was. As a high-risk patient, he wanted my LDL at less than 70; and for that reason, he wanted to increase my cholesterol medicine again. I thought, *"Here we go again."* I was less than thrilled, but I knew I needed to give it a try in order to bring the numbers closer in line with where they needed to be. He was going to increase it from 10 milligrams to 40 milligrams. I winced and reminded him of my past issues, we then settled on 20 milligrams. He said that if that didn't work, we could try the 10 milligram statin along with another type of cholesterol medication that worked in the digestive track. At least we had a plan-B, just in case.

I haven't received any other explanation from my doctor as to the cause of my symptoms. Still though, I perceive he's not convinced that the issues that I have experienced are statin related. He feels if it were the statins causing the problems, that I would be feeling the effects in other parts of my body as well, not just the chest. I *suppose* that could be the case, perhaps there is another reason for my symptoms. On the other hand, the "statin holidays" that I have taken, followed by a rechallenge of different statins, have persuaded *me* into thinking that they *were* the cause. Other than my LDL not being lower, my doctor felt like I was doing great. I did too, now all I needed to do was to work at getting my LDL down.

It was such a relief to be feeling better, not perfect, but better. I didn't expect a miracle, I just wanted to feel normal again to be able to just live my life ... to be able to live my life without worrying if in the next moment something was going to change and turn my life upside down again. I didn't think that was too much to ask. Only *another* heart attack survivor would understand how these numerous setbacks, even small ones, negatively affect you. Everything seems to be looking up and then a setback happens. You worry that the positive outcome that you were counting on might only be *wishful thinking*. As time has gone by, I've come to realize what may have seemed like *setbacks* at the time, were just a normal part of the recovery process. It's just hard to deal with when you have been through such a traumatic event. It would seem that the emotional toll is sometimes more difficult to overcome than the physical one. I knew though, I was at this point, feeling stronger emotionally. Looking back with the aid of hindsight, I realize now that many of my fears *were not* rational. Nonetheless, that *did not* make them any less unsettling during those difficult moments.

The one-year anniversary of my heart attack was nearing. With *all* the research I had done it stated that the first year was the most crucial. I wanted and *needed* that one-year mark to come. I guess that I felt if only I could make it to that mark, then I would be okay.

CHAPTER 33

Nearly a year had gone by since that *life-altering* day. I've reflected back on *many* things and one of those things has been the fact that I didn't take cholesterol medications for all those years when I needed it. If you will remember, while I was still in the hospital, I was at first angry with myself over that. Even though I know *now* that it *was* one of the big contributors toward my heart disease, with the aid of retrospection I am able to see things from a different perspective. I have forgiven myself for that error in judgment especially in light of all the problems I have had with those types of medications. The reason I say this is because I know myself, if I had agreed to take the medication years ago and started to have issues with it, I would have most likely stopped taking it. I may have tried a second time, but in all probability, *not*. The bottom line is, in all likelihood, I wouldn't have continued taking cholesterol medication.

Since I was unable to foresee what was ahead, why beat myself up over it now? What's done is done, in the past and can't be changed. However, I do at present have the power and knowledge to change my future. I have *proven to myself* that I really do need it and I take it *faithfully* now.

There are *many* factors that have contributed toward my successful recovery. In spite of the issues that I have had with *some* of them, one factor I feel *was* my medications. I know that's probably *not* what you expected me to say, it just took some trial and error to find the *right* ones for me. While I was in the hospital nearly everyone that I spoke with, stressed the importance of taking my medication and taking it correctly, and I feel finally finding the *right* ones have played a major role in my recovery process.

In my journey, I observed that the majority of people don't know very much about the medications they take on a daily basis. Most can tell you the color and perhaps the shape, but little else. I have a suggestion for anyone out there who takes any type of medication, especially long term. First, learn the names of all of your regular medications. Learn the brand name as well as the generic name because at times medical professionals will use either name interchangeably. Next, it's good to know the *reason* you are taking that particular medication. What is its purpose? All prescriptions come with an information sheet when they are filled. Read it *carefully* in order to be aware of side effects and possible food or drug interactions. It's also helpful to know the *class* that your drug belongs to since the information sheet will sometimes only list the class of drug when warning of a possible interaction. As I read the information sheet, I highlight the side effects and keep it handy in order to refer back to it. Make a list of all of your medications, including strengths and dosages and include medications to which you are allergic. Keep this list *updated* and with you at *all times*. You may even want to give a copy to a close family member or friend, just in case.

August 15, 2012
The one-year anniversary of my heart attack

A day *so long* in arriving, a day I once feared I may *never* see. No, I ate no cake to celebrate, but I did give a lot of thought as to how I should remember this special occasion. I am truly grateful for how far I've come, and I appreciate that a great deal of my health success is largely due to the excellent medical care that I received. It was because of that fact, on this anniversary occasion, I took the time to write a special thank you note to both of my cardiologists. I wanted to express my gratitude to them for helping me to get to this milestone. I delivered it to their office along with a box of my *pre-heart attack favorite* cookies. In case you're wondering, they were *not* heart healthy cookies, and no, I didn't eat any. I just wanted them to know how much I appreciated the part they played in giving me a second chance at the rest of my life. I am more confident now than *ever* that you can't keep a strong Cajun woman down, at least not for very long. We *are* a determined breed!

How do I feel now a year along? Overall, I feel good and whole again. There *is* truth to the old adage, what doesn't kill you makes you stronger. When I think about it, there isn't even one thing that I was able to do before the heart attack that I can't do now. It just may take a little more time and effort to do it now. I will probably never be able to climb Mount Everest, but I never had plans to do that anyway. Despite the way I felt in the beginning, I now know there *is* life after a heart attack! It can be a good life if it's met with the right attitude and we surround ourselves with people who love us. Believe me; a year can make a tremendous difference! It's amazing to me that I came from what *felt* like the brink of death, to where I am today.

I occasionally have some tightness in my chest, as well as sporadic shortness of breath, but it's not *nearly* to the degree that it has been in the past. I think I may still need an adjustment or two in my medication. We are not quite there yet, but we *will* eventually get it right. I can never forget that I am a cardiac patient, even if I wanted to forget, I'm reminded at least twice everyday when I have to take my medications. This is just part of my life from here on out. I consider it a small price to pay for my health.

I know I'm more paranoid (I mean that figuratively, not as a clinical diagnosis.) *now*, than I was before the heart attack. Nevertheless, I'm not *nearly* as paranoid as I was shortly after the heart attack. Facing your own mortality will change you. When you've experienced such a traumatic event in your life, you cannot, *not* take notice of a flutter or a twinge in your chest without trepidations. I've talked to others who have been through similar experiences and they've told me they feel the same way. You're just a little more conscious of what is going on inside of you because you gain a certain awareness that you didn't take notice of before. You are more in-tune with listening to what your body is trying to tell you. Overall, I know that I'm in a better place both physically and emotionally than I was a year ago. I recently heard a quote that stated, "Nothing makes you want to live more than being close to death." It is *so* true!

I do wish I had more energy, as stated previously, that has *always* been an issue for me. Of course, I am a year older; I guess that probably has something to do with it too. I don't have the stamina I would like to have and mornings continue to be a real *challenge* for me. It takes much more effort on my part just to get going. I don't like being tired, but I have learned when I'm tired, I have to rest. It's just that simple. There are no restrictions on my physical activity. If I feel like I can do it, I do.

Over this year, I have lost thirty pounds. I would guess I'm at an average weight for my height now. A person recently referred to me as tall and slim. I thought they were talking to someone else. It had been a long time since anyone had said that. The weight loss and the fact that I lost my hot flashes are two big benefits. Now, I eat a good, balanced, heart healthy diet and try to watch my portion size. I have to be honest though, sometimes that does get old. At times, I would like to "pig out" on something that I really enjoy eating. I do indulge occasionally in some treat, but I try to return to healthy eating, right away. In doing this, I don't feel like I'm being deprived. I feel this is important because eating this way *has* to be a way of life for me now. Another benefit I have experienced would be that my blood sugar levels are much better now than before. In fact, during my last visit with my endocrinologist he told me, with the improvements I've made, he may not even still classify me as pre-diabetic. He said he felt I was in better general health now than before the heart attack. I was thrilled to hear this news and realized something else. I came to the conclusion that a heart healthy lifestyle isn't *only* heart-smart; it benefits other organs of the entire body as well. For instance, a heart healthy diet not only lowers cholesterol that can lead to plaque build-up in the arteries of the heart, it can lower the plaques ability to form clots that can break off. This is helpful in lowering your risk for stroke, so that is of benefit to the brain. Not smoking is good for the heart as well as your lungs. Watching your fats and alcohol intake is beneficial to your liver. Restricting salt intake is good for the kidneys and blood pressure. Limiting carbs (especially simple carbs) is good for your pancreas and weight loss. *And*, staying physically active is good not only for weight loss but just good *overall* well being. All these other things will come as a bonus to good heart health.

One of the negative aspects I have noticed is a change in my skin. I know that some of it has to do with my weight loss and some I feel is my medication. My skin seems to have a different texture; it's much more delicate and fragile now. I can see in the mirror too, that this ordeal has definitely aged me. I don't like that either, but that too is something else I cannot change. Again, in this regard, *I am a year older*. There is one thing regarding my skin that has changed for the better. I have Rosacea and have noticed a dramatic improvement in this condition. I think that this may also have something to do with the medications I take as well.

Another thing that I deal with is bruising; this is one of the side effects of the anti-platelet medication. Most of the time, when I notice a bruise, I can't even recall what caused it. I've counted as many as twenty-two bruises on my body on a single occasion. I understand that in time, I may be able to stop taking it, but my cardiologist will decide when that will happen.

On one occasion, someone referred to me as a "heart attack victim." I don't feel like that was an accurate reference. I was a heart attack victim the morning that it occurred. However, every single moment since then, I have proudly been a heart attack *survivor*!

When I think about how far I have come since that night of being admitted to the hospital, I feel it's truly remarkable because I have made tremendous progress. I feel *very blessed* in this regard and try not to take *anything* for granted. I'm thankful and grateful to be a part of *each* new day. It continues to be challenging, but I *try* to lead a calm, happy life. Proverbs 14:30 tells us, "A calm heart gives life to the body." The Creator of the physical heart knows what is best for us, and I *thank* him each and every day for this wonderful gift of life.

You may wonder specifically why I decided to write this story. Please allow me to share my reasons for this undertaking. Several months after my heart attack, I had gone to visit my daughter in New Orleans. I expressed to her that I was very tired. My daughter asked if I hadn't slept well the night before. I told her, no that I hadn't.

I said to her, "I have a hard time going to sleep *every* night, because I replay my heart attack over and over in my head."

The memories were so unpleasant; it was as if they were *seared* into my brain. I found remembering to be painful and consuming, nevertheless, in some strange way, I was almost *afraid* to forget. My daughter made the suggestion if I would write down what had happened to me, maybe that would help me to deal with it. I casually told her that might work and I would consider it. At that moment though, I wasn't giving it any *serious* consideration. However, I continued to mull over the idea for the next few weeks. Then one day as I was thinking about what she had proposed, I decided that I would take her suggestion. I had plenty going on that day, but I sat down and wrote the first two pages. I didn't go back to it for about a week. I would just write a *little* whenever I had some extra time. I didn't want to tell a soul at first because I was unsure if I could remember enough to create a complete story. As I continued to write, I was surprised at how much and how many details I did remember, *that* made me want to write more.

This project started as a catharsis to help me heal. I was just going to write an abbreviated version to start with, just a few notes scribbled down. As I continued to remember details and put them down in writing, I first thought, "I might have a short story on my hands." As I wrote even more I thought, "Is it *possible* that I could write a book?" As the pages were filling up, my purpose for this project was *evolving*, my thoughts *now* were, "Maybe, besides helping myself, I might actually be able to help someone else by putting my thoughts and feelings on paper. Maybe I can pay this forward." The more I worked on this project the more I wanted to. In time, I could *hardly* wait to get to the computer to write. However, I had no background or experience in writing. It had been more years than I care to mention since I had taken an English class. So, I just wrote from the "heart" and *this* is what came out. If someone had told me that I would one day write a book, I would have laughed and thought they were out of their minds. This was never a goal of mine; *this* was something that *other* people accomplish. I thought only people, who are really smart, funny, or interesting, wrote books, not this little ole Cajun girl.

As I have worked on this project, I've had to play these events over in my head. Remember, *that* was the problem originally. It did bring back many unpleasant memories and feelings. However, replaying it for this purpose has been *different* somehow. It seems that putting it on paper gets it out of my head and into a place where it can help someone else. I once read, to off-load anxieties by putting them down on paper, frees you to focus on the tasks that are in front of you. This is evidently true. I recommend this therapeutic exercise to anyone dealing with any emotional event in his or her life. As I write this, I don't know if it will ever be published. I don't know if anyone besides my family and friends will ever read it. I can live with that because I know how cathartic writing this has been for me. It has helped me to deal with my inner self too and I'm able to see my heart attack in a different light. I was able to *analyze* and *explore* all my thoughts and feelings *at my own pace*. That has enabled me to put the entire ordeal into a perspective that I could live with *and* move forward with my life. It has helped me as well to come to terms with the answers to my many, many questions. It has helped me learn a lot about myself too. In his memoirs, Dan Rather said, "In writing a book, you find out things about yourself that you didn't know." That is so true, and I have learned other things through this process that I would like to share with you.

I have learned that you can have *major* blockages and not know it.

I have learned that you can have symptoms that come and go over extended periods of time. Just because the symptoms *seem* to go away doesn't necessarily mean you're okay.

I have learned just because you *think* you are in good health, doesn't mean you are; also just because you *want* to be, doesn't mean you will be.

I have learned that ignoring the facts *will not* change them (don't be an ostrich).

I have learned genetics play a *HUGE* role in our health.

I have learned that neither age, nor gender matter, heart attacks *are not* selective.

I have learned when your cholesterol is high, *don't* ignore it.

I have learned when your doctor tells you something, (such as, you need cholesterol meds) sometimes they just *may* know better, even if you think you do. I think the majority of doctors have our best interests at heart.

I have learned that we *know* our own bodies and can, for the most part, sense when there is something wrong (even if we aren't sure what). If your doctor won't listen to you, *continue* searching until you find a doctor who will listen and take you seriously.

I have learned that a heart attack *doesn't* mean that your life is over. There is hope for a full recovery, no matter how fragile and *"crumpled"* you feel at the time. You *can* feel whole again!

I have learned the heart *can* heal very quickly, given the right circumstances, and provided you heed your doctor's advice.

I have learned that heart disease *does not* define you. Only you, the inner person, can define *you*.

I have learned the *earlier* you accept the things that you cannot change, the more contented you will be in life.

I have learned that despite the seriousness of the circumstances, it's *best* to try to keep your sense of humor. People who laugh a lot tend to live longer.

I have learned that even in bad circumstances *good things* can come out of it, even if it's only a new awareness or attitude.

I've learned it is best not to dwell on what you didn't do, that's unproductive. You can't change the past, but you can alter your future. Dwell on your future with a positive attitude.

And *finally*, I have learned that having a loving family and friends are the *very best* medicine of all for your heart!

Let's Have a Heart To Heart Talk

As I did research for this book, I read and learned many important and interesting facts about the heart. Even though a number of these facts may not have been a part of my personal story, I feel I would be remiss not to include some of them. People (and specifically women) need to know these things in order to be proactive about their heart health. My observations are aimed specifically at women, but much of this applies to men as well.

It's quite funny; it seems by default, I have now become the so-called "expert" on heart related matters. When someone has a question, it seems that I am the one to call. I have even had a total stranger call and say, "You don't know me, but I'm a friend of so-in-so. Would you mind if I ask you a few questions about your heart attack?" I tell people what I know on a personal level. What one has to keep in mind though, just as a man's heart attack is different from that of a woman, even a woman's heart attack varies from woman *to* woman. There are *no* "cookie cutter" symptoms to rely on. I always remind anyone asking for advice that I have no medical training. If they are having ANY *real issues*, I whole-heartedly (no pun intended) encourage them to see a cardiologist. *Do not* try to diagnose this yourself, because delaying can exact a very high cost. While in actuality I am no expert, I am *now* an advocate for the importance of heart health.

I considered calling this appendix "Heart Trivia." Nevertheless, there is *nothing* trivial about this strong muscle that beats two billion, 500 million times in a lifetime and circulates approximately 1800 gallons of blood (in women) throughout the body daily. While I embarked on my self-taught, "Cardiology for Dummies 101" course, I was totally amazed and awed at the things I was learning about this marvelous, complex organ. Nonetheless, this marvelous, complex organ needs protecting. One of the primary ways that we can protect our hearts is by being aware of our individual risk factors. In many cases, this is where it all starts. A heart attack can result from years or maybe even *decades* of risks associated with one or more risk factors. We've all heard, "To be forewarned is to be forearmed." Learning our risk factors can help us to specifically fight the ones that apply personally. This will help us to be more vigilant so that we can take the proper steps to modify our lives and life styles in order to reduce our risk for heart disease. There are two categories of risk factors; there are those that we *can* and those that we *cannot* control. Let's consider the latter first.

Inherited (genetic) Risk Factors:

Gender- Generally, men under age 50 are more at risk than women of the same age group. A woman's risk increases after menopause, due to the sharp decrease in the hormone, estrogen.

Increasing Age- A woman's risk for heart disease increases as she ages. Woman usually have heart attacks at older ages than men do, this is one reason that women are more likely to die from a heart attack. However, younger women can and do experience heart attacks.

Heredity- There is a greater risk of developing heart disease if a close blood relative is affected by it, especially if it occurs before the age of 55. However, even though you are born with certain risk factors, they can be improved with life style changes and medical management. Just because it's in our genetics doesn't mean we are doomed; it should be our wake-up call to be more alert. Some give in to their genetics, feeling that genetic predisposition is something impossible to fight. I've arrived at one conclusion on this matter. Unless we have had extensive genetic testing, we don't know *specifically* what genetic markers we carry. Even then, we can't be *exactly* sure how those markers will affect us personally. When I think about my own risk factors, I attribute my heart disease mainly to heredity and high cholesterol. I had no control over my genetics, but I *could* have had some control over my high cholesterol. However, I made the erroneous choice not to take cholesterol medications. What if perhaps my *only* genetic marker for heart disease, was to have a predisposition toward high cholesterol? Had I not ignored my high cholesterol, it may *not* have been a contributing factor towards my heart attack. I know this is speculative on my part, but my point is—we have to fight these risk factors in *every* way possible. At the very least, we will be improving our odds for a healthier heart. We will also have fewer regrets, knowing that we did *all* we could.

Ethnicity- Certain ethnic groups are at greater risk for heart disease than others are. For example, African American women are at greater risk for heart disease than Caucasian women are. Telling your doctor your ethnic background may help him to better estimate your heart disease risk.

Previous Heart Attack- Women who have had a heart attack are at greater risk for a second heart attack. Twenty-two percent of women aged 40-69 who survive a first heart attack will have another within five years. This is why we have to remain vigilant in our care, post-MI.

High Cholesterol- Of course, I know firsthand the part that this risk plays in heart disease. This risk factor can probably fit into both risk categories. While our bodies need a certain amount of cholesterol, *too much* can be detrimental to our health. Produced in the liver, the blood carries cholesterol to our cells, in molecules called lipoproteins. There are low-density lipoproteins (LDL) and high-density lipoproteins (HDL). When there is too much LDL cholesterol (our bad cholesterol) concentrated in the blood, the cholesterol becomes a risk factor for coronary artery disease. HDL (our good cholesterol) is thought to play a protective role by removing cholesterol from tissues and carrying it back to the liver where it is altered and eliminated from the body. If LDL is high and HDL is low, this increases your risk for heart disease. Your risk may drop when you lower your LDL levels. This can be done with diet, exercise, and medication. A woman's total cholesterol levels and triglycerides tend to rise after menopause.

Acquired Risk Factors:

We can have some control over these by making changes and modifying our lifestyle. Keeping the acquired risk factors under control can make the genetic risk factors less of a threat. When you change your lifestyle, it's possible to modify your genes. You may turn off the bad genes and turn on the good genes.

Diet- By eating a balanced, heart-healthy diet, we can lower our risk factor. Eat a diet that is low in saturated fats and free of trans fats. Make it rich in fresh vegetables and fruits. Include high fiber foods, whole grains, and lean protein. The addition of fish, specifically those high in omega-3 fatty acids are very beneficial. Limit the amount of carbohydrates because too many carbs may raise your triglyceride levels. Strictly limit your intake of sodium, red and cured meats as well.

Sedentary Life-Style- Heart disease has been shown to be twice as prevalent in people who are inactive. Even simple exercise such as brisk walking for 20-30 minutes on most days of the week can make a *real* difference. Regular exercise strengthens your heart and improves the heart's ability to pump. It improves circulation and helps your body use oxygen more efficiently. Added benefits are it aids in weight loss, as well as lowering cholesterol and blood pressure. Exercise can improve *all other* risk factors. Even if you hate to exercise, view it as another form of "medication" that you do for your heart. The added benefit is you will feel better too. The American Heart Association says that for *each* hour of physical activity you engage in, you'll add about two hours of life expectancy—even if you don't start until middle age. Physical activity is *anything* in which you move your body and burn calories. If you have been sedentary for a long time, work up slowly towards your goal by increasing your time, as you get stronger.

Smoking- Smoking is responsible for 50% of the heart attacks in women under age 55. It is the *single most preventable* cause of heart attack. Prolonged exposure to secondhand smoke also increases your risk. Smoking increases blood pressure and introduces toxic chemicals like nicotine and carbon monoxide into the blood stream. These chemicals have been shown to damage your arteries. If you smoke, stop *NOW*!

High Blood Pressure- High blood pressure damages artery walls and allows LDL cholesterol to enter the artery lining. This in turn, promotes the buildup of plaque. As these plaque deposits buildup there is more restriction of blood flow, which causes an elevation in blood pressure. For every one-point decrease in the diastolic pressure, the risk of a heart attack may be reduced by 2 to 3 percent.

Excess Weight- Obesity is a major risk factor for many different disorders. It can put you at higher risk for such things as heart disease, high cholesterol, high blood pressure, diabetes, and stroke. Persons who are overweight by 30% or more, are at greater risk. Dr. Oz says that gaining even 20 pounds, increases your risk factor. He says that our body type can also play a role, stressing the risks involved in having excess belly fat.

Diabetes- Diabetes accelerates cardiovascular disease and increases the risk for heart attack. In fact, you are two to four times more likely to die from heart disease if you have uncontrolled diabetes. Avoiding obesity is one of the ways you may prevent diabetes. People with diabetes often have high blood pressure and elevated cholesterol levels as well. Diabetics tend to have smaller, denser LDL particles that are more likely to cause cardiovascular damage.

Stress- A person who is under serious stress is at greater risk for heart attack and sudden cardiac death. Stress can cause the arteries to constrict and if there is plaque buildup in those arteries, this will greatly reduce the blood flow to the coronary arteries causing an increased workload on your heart. Prolonged stress can even create the environment for plaque in artery walls to rupture. Chronic anger and hostility can raise blood pressure, increase the heart rate, and stimulate the liver to dump cholesterol into the bloodstream. This damages coronary arteries and contributes to coronary artery disease. Anger and stress are sometimes just a part of life; however, how we deal with it is what is important. *Intense* anger is thought to double the heart attack risk, and this remains an immediate danger for at least two hours.

Alcohol Use- People who drink *excessive* amounts of alcohol on a regular basis are at greater risk for heart disease. Drink alcohol only in moderation, no more than one drink daily for women or two drinks for a man.

Periodontal Disease- The jury is still out on this one and there are conflicting opinions about a causative link between gum disease and heart disease. In the past, the development of heart disease has been *directly* linked to poor dental hygiene. It was thought that bacteria in the mouth related to gum disease, move into the bloodstream and cause inflammation in the blood vessels, thereby contributing to heart disease. However, in a recent statement from the American Heart Association, they say there is insufficient evidence to *prove* that gum disease causes atherosclerotic heart disease. What we do know is gum disease and heart disease both produces markers of inflammation such as C-reactive protein, and chronic inflammation *is* linked to heart disease. While no *direct* connection has *yet* been made, why chance it? Regular dental care, daily brushing and flossing is *always* a good idea whether it's good for your heart or not.

Pregnancy Complications - This one may surprise you as much as it did me. In my research, I discovered that pregnancy-related hypertensive disorders such as preeclampsia and gestational diabetes were linked to an increased risk for heart disease later in life. Pregnancy has been compared to a nine-month stress test because of the increased workload on the body. If you "fail the test" by developing complications, you may find yourself at greater risk for heart disease. This is not because the pregnancy complications caused the problem, but rather because it revealed the problem. Interestingly, I had pre-eclampsia thirty-one years earlier with my first child.

The best way to protect ourselves from coronary artery disease is to prevent it from happening in the first place. Know your numbers (blood pressure, glucose, cholesterol, BMI, and waist circumference) and have them checked *regularly*. By applying the preceding suggestions, and changing the things that we *do* have control over, we can make a tremendous difference in our heart and overall health.

***

Warning Signs of a Heart Attack

Please don't discount my advice about the warning signs of a heart attack. I know I missed the symptoms of my own heart attack, but I have learned volumes in the last year. I am now far removed from that woman who at times foolishly ignored her heart health.

I learned that the location of the pain might depend on the area of the heart affected. Sometimes it's not just one type of pain, but it may be a *composite* of several different symptoms. These symptoms can manifest themselves in many different forms. A woman's symptoms are sometimes vaguer and less impressive than a man's symptoms and at times they don't even present all at once. These variations are probably what lead women to deny and dismiss what they are feeling. We try to convince ourselves that what we are feeling is just normal aches and pains, when that is *not* the case. For this reason, women take longer than men do, to react to the warning signs of a heart attack. With time at a premium, this delays the start of life-saving treatment at such a critical time. The majority of persons who have a heart attack survive if they arrive at the hospital alive, but the overall outcome is better the earlier that treatment can be initiated. **Do not** hesitate to seek medical attention. Your very life depends on getting medical intervention as soon as possible. Even if you are unsure, ***it is better to be wrong about your symptoms and be alive.***

About six months after my heart attack, I watched an episode of Dr. Oz dealing with the warning signs of a woman's heart attack. Needless to say, I watched my mentor with rapt attention. I wanted to know where I had gone wrong. The following is *my* analysis of what he said that day. The first warning sign he talked about was neck, shoulder, and jaw pain. I had all of these for two weeks prior to my heart attack. Dr. Oz said, to pay particular attention to pain that radiates down the arm; I had that too. It can be pain anywhere in the upper body. He also advised, to time the pain. Does it last longer than one minute? If it does, it may be heart related. He also recommended doing the pinpoint test. Can you pinpoint the pain with the tip of your finger? If you cannot do this, it may be your heart. Heart related pain much of the time is associated with activity. You should also be aware that besides pain, there might be pressure, heaviness or a squeezing feeling that is not fleeting.

He next talked about gastrointestinal symptoms such as nausea, indigestion, and stomach pain. He said if you take anti-acids and your symptoms do not go away, it could possibly be heart related. I understand that some people also experience vomiting.

Subsequently, he referred to shortness of breath as a symptom. Are you experiencing shortness of breath while performing normal daily activities? Can you breathe normally and talk while you walk? If not, it may be a symptom of a heart related issue.

The next symptom that he discussed was dizziness or lightheadedness. Lightheadedness occurs when your blood pressure drops too low. Dr. Oz said that when these other warning signs and/or chest pain accompany it, we should take notice. Ask yourself these questions. Am I dizzy while sitting? (You should not be.) Does it go away?

He then discussed the symptom of unusual fatigue— an *overwhelming* feeling of exhaustion. He said that

70% of women have unusual fatigue in the days or weeks leading up to the heart attack. Ask yourself, is there a change in the daily activities of my life? Can I perform those activities without needing to take a rest? You can compare last year's activities to see if there has been a big difference.

There are a few other symptoms that I would like to include. These as well, *should not be ignored.*
If a person feels any of the preceding or following symptoms, either alone or in combination with other symptoms, you should seek medical attention promptly.

- Severe pressure, tightness, fullness or squeezing pain across or centered in the chest that lasts more than a few minutes
- Weakness, profuse sweating, clammy feeling skin, paleness or fainting
- An impending feeling of doom or sudden general feeling of illness
- Headache and/or blurry vision
- Heart palpitations, rapid or irregular heartbeat
- Chest or back pain that increases in intensity and that is not relieved by nitroglycerin or rest

Ask yourself, does this feel different from what I've experienced before? Is the discomfort stronger or lasting longer than usual? *The bottom line is ... if you are in doubt, get it checked out.* Only **YOU** have the power to discern your symptoms and *beat* the number one killer of women. The good news is you don't have to wait for these symptoms to arise. There are simple life-saving tests that can help diagnose a problem, even before there are symptoms.

One test that can help to predict heart disease is the CRP test. CRP stands for C-reactive protein. This test scores the level of inflammation in our bodies. The more inflammation in our body likely means more plaque; it's the body's way of trying to sooth the inflammation. Because of this, elevated CRP levels can be a predictor of cardiovascular disease. This is based on its correlation with the other known cardiac risk factors. An elevated CRP level puts you at 4 times more risk for a heart attack or stroke.

A level of less than one is the lowest level of risk. A level that is between 1.0-3.0 is considered average. Levels that are higher than 3.0 are considered to be at the highest risk. However, women with a level of 2.7 or higher are at twice the risk for a heart attack or stroke. Women with a 3.0 level or higher are at a four times greater risk. It's ironic that shortly before my heart attack; I had read about this test and had planned to ask my endocrinologist to order this test for me. I am very curious as to what it would have showed.

Dr. Oz also recommends an LDL particle size test. If you have a predominance of the larger, "fluffy" LDL particles, you are at a lower risk for plaque build-up. This is because larger LDL particles are not as likely to embed into the artery walls. A predominance of the small, dense LDL particles puts you at a higher risk for coronary artery disease progression.

Dr. Oz spoke of a simple and free test that we can perform at home. He called it the "stretch test." To perform the test you are to bend over and touch your toes without bouncing. He said the farther that you could stretch; the more flexible your arteries tend to be. Stretching exercises increases the flexibility of your arteries. He recommended doing stretching exercises for 30 minutes, 3 times a week.

Another simple, free test is to check your pulse. A woman's average resting heart rate should be between 60-80 beats per minute. If your resting heart rate is *consistently* above 90, the chance of dying from heart disease is 3 times higher than if the rate is 60-80.

He also spoke about the waist/hip ratio. This test is to more accurately determine belly fat. Divide the waist measurement by the hip measurement. This number should be less than .85 for women. He said that this test is more accurate than body mass index for determining belly fat.

***

Now, you have recognized that *something* is wrong. You surmise that you are *possibly* having a heart attack, *what* do you do now? Action steps are now required. Do not try to wait to see if the symptoms will go away. If you are in reality having a heart attack, surviving may depend on getting medical attention as soon as possible. Stop what you are doing and sit or lie down. Loosen any tight clothing or belts. If you're having difficulty breathing, sitting semi-upright may be a position that is more comfortable. Call 911 and tell the dispatcher that you suspect that you are having a heart attack. Try to remain *calm* and breathe *deeply* and *slowly*.

Many medical professionals recommend that you *chew* an aspirin at the *onset* of symptoms. Chewing the aspirin allows the medicine to be absorbed more quickly than swallowing it whole. Some persons are unable to take aspirin, so check with your doctor in advance on this. If your doctor has prescribed nitrates for you, take them as directed at the onset of symptoms. If you have access to oxygen, use it.

If you are around family or out in public, make *someone* aware that you think you *may* be having a heart attack. In this way others can render assistance, perhaps even give CPR if your condition gets worse. If you are alone, call someone who lives nearby and can arrive the quickest, like a neighbor. Tell them that you think you are having a heart attack, and have taken aspirin. Unlock your door and wait near the front door.

If you are in an isolated location, or if it will take paramedics a long time to reach you, have someone drive you to the hospital. Remember though, if you call for an ambulance, an EMT will likely begin treatment while en route to the hospital. **Do *not*** try to drive yourself because of the risk of having an accident. In the meanwhile, try to remain calm and minimize your activity. If you are driving at the time that you experience symptoms, pull over and flag someone down or call 911 and wait for paramedics to arrive.

None of us plans on having a serious medical emergency. However, there is something that we can do in advance, that will help us, if we do have one. As I spoke about earlier, everyone should carry in their wallet, an *updated* list of his or her medications and the medications to which they are allergic. This will help the emergency room staff to properly and safely treat you. In an emergency situation, you *may not* remember these medications. *This is very important*!

Our bodies are wonderfully made; we just need to be in tune with what it is trying to tell us. We use our instincts and *woman's intuition* for many things; use it for this purpose too. Deep down inside we usually know when something is wrong, even if we aren't sure what.

This is because we know our bodies better than anyone else does.

Unfortunately, sometimes even our doctors aren't quite convinced that we, as women, are in fact having a heart attack. This is because a woman's symptoms are much of the time, atypical. Sadly, women are all too often dismissed or misdiagnosed, and some *don't survive*. My recommendation is to be direct and assert yourself! *Insist* that your doctor take you seriously and listen to you. My mother has always said, "The wheel that squeaks the loudest is the one that will get the grease."

The bottom line is we have to be our *own* first line of defense in our heart health. We cannot make the mistake of thinking that this just happens to someone else. Be proactive about your heart health, think—"*prevent and protect*" in the lifestyle choices made. To a large extent, heart disease is preventable, but it requires a focused effort and diligence on our part. Nevertheless, to paraphrase the hair color ad, "We're worth it."

In conclusion, I hope I have shown that our heart attacks can be as unique and different as we are. Our symptoms can vary from mild to strong and do not occur in the same manner with every heart attack *or* with every person. I was extremely fortunate that my eventual outcome was as good as it was, considering that my treatment was delayed for such a long time. I was the *exception*, not the rule! My advice is *don't* dismiss those advance warning signs, they're *trying* to tell you something. Acting early can prevent needless heart damage. I ask you to *please* learn from my mistakes.

You *can* take an active role in saving your own life! We only get one heart, sometimes we only get *one chance* to save it ... *don't* blow that chance.

Be a survivor!

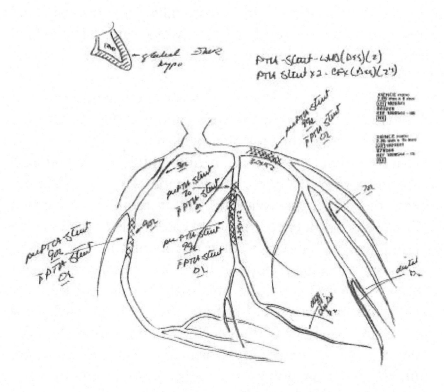

This is a diagram of the coronary arteries of my heart. The X's are where the stents are placed. The artery on the far left is the RCA (90% blockage). The one in the middle is the CIRC (there are two stents in the CIRC-70% and 99% blockages) and the one on the far right is the LAD (99% blockage).

E-Mail address:
Cajunheartattack@yahoo.com

Watch the Videos
www.youtube.com/watch?v=6Fu3I6IXsPs
www.youtube.com/watch?v=zKKiP9q04C8
www.youtube.com/watch?v=vNt2npXtw5I
(Case sensitive)

EBR

3 2400 039845395